Nursing in Primary Health Care

Nursing in Primary Health Care offers a fresh and rigorous approach to the important issues facing nurses both now and in the future. It analyses recent policy changes, assesses their effect on the delivery of health and social care in the community, and explores the challenges they represent for nurses.

The opening chapter, 'Policy overview', provides a clear and detailed background to the practice issues dealt with in the rest of the book. These include assessment strategies; the importance of working across professional and agency boundaries; setting standards and defining outcomes in the quest for a high-quality and cost-effective service; the needs of carers as well as clients. Taking into account the new nursing roles which are emerging in response to changing health care needs, Fiona Ross and Ann Mackenzie review the appropriate use of skills and challenge accepted ways of working.

Suitable for undergraduate and postgraduate studies in community nursing and for students following Project 2000 diploma courses, *Nursing in Primary Health Care* encourages a questioning approach to policy and the consequences of its implementation.

Fiona Ross is Professor of Primary Care Nursing at St George's Hospital Medical School, London. **Ann Mackenzie** is Professor of Clinical Nursing at The Chinese University of Hong Kong.

Nursing in Primary Health Care

Policy into Practice

Fiona Ross and Ann Mackenzie

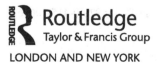

Routledge
Taylor & Francis Group

LONDON AND NEW YORK

First published 1996
by Routledge
2 Park Square, Milton Park, Abingdon, Oxon, OX14 4RN
605 Third Avenue, New York, NY 10017

*Routledge is an imprint of the Taylor & Francis Group, an
informa business*

© 1996 Fiona Ross and Ann Mackenzie

Typeset in Times by
Florencetype Ltd, Stoodleigh, Devon

British Library Cataloguing in Publication Data
A catalogue record for this book is available from
the British Library

Library of Congress Cataloguing in Publication Data
A catalogue record for this book has been requested

ISBN 13: 978-0-415-10616-0 (pbk)

Contents

Illustrations

Boxes

Figures

Tables

Acknowledgements

The authors would like to thank the following for their valuable contributions to the successful completion of this book:

Terry Mackenzie for his discerning reading and editing of the final typescript and his support throughout.

John Tatam and our children Hannah, Hugo and Jonny for their forbearance.

Margaret Elliott for researching and collating innovations in community nursing practice specially for this book.

Dr Christina Victor, Senior Lecturer in Public Health in the Department of Public Health Sciences at St George's Hospital Medical School, London University, for Chapter 2, 'Health-needs profiling'.

Introduction

The role and scope of nursing in primary health care is continually evolving as a result of changes in society. The aim of this book is to explore and discuss current and important issues in primary health and community care from the perspective of nursing. The authors recognise that the frame of nursing in primary care is changing rapidly. It is anticipated that change will be continuous, and to some extent unpredictable. Therefore the emphasis of this book will be on exploring current trends, tensions and dilemmas underlying the pressures for change in primary health care nursing. It does not aim to be a comprehensive text; rather to analyse, interpret and explain how policy informs practice, drawing from a number of disciplines including sociology, epidemiology, social policy and nursing. The in-depth appraisal of important contemporary issues draws on published research and examples from practice to inform practitioners, educators, managers and researchers and to offer a questioning approach to policy information and the consequences of implementation in practice.

The interest in nursing in primary health care comes from our professional experience in district nursing, as well as our teaching and research in an increasingly wider arena including health visiting, practice nursing and general practice. We recognise that the boundaries between nursing disciplines in the community are shifting as the internal market and new approaches to primary health care develop. We have therefore chosen to focus this book as far as possible on generic nursing issues in the primary health care setting. This is in order to avoid becoming trapped by the unfortunate, but familiar, territorialism that often preoccupies district nursing, health visiting and practice nursing, which on

the whole fuels concerns only of professional status rather than
of patient care. Some may say that this approach is the fore-
runner to the slippery slope of advocating a generic nurse for
primary health care. It is clear to us that there are distinct roles
in community nursing, but that as a group they face shared and
common challenges, and in order to understand these it is helpful
to take a common approach.

Definitions

Primary health care. There are various definitions of primary
health care. There is the elaborate and somewhat idealistic
definition from the World Health Organisation that defines
primary health care as essential care based on practical, scientific-
ally sound and acceptable methods and technology, made
universally available to individuals and families in the community
through their full participation and at a cost that community and
country can afford and maintain at every stage of their development in the spirit of self-reliance and self-determination (WHO
1978a). These objectives, although laudable, perhaps lose some
of their significance, because of the attempt to be universal and
thus relevant for societies in the West as well as the East,
for countries with developed and complex health systems and for
those countries where the struggle is about nutrition and safe water
supplies.

In the report *New World, New Opportunities* (NHSME 1993a),
primary health care is described as the first point of contact for
people seeking advice, support and treatment. It outlines the
responsibilities of primary health care to allow and encourage
people to participate in the planning and organisation and
management of their own health care at home, school, work and
in the GP practice. It includes health surveillance, health promotion, acute episodic and continuing care.

Primary health care nurses are defined by the above report
as those nurses working outside hospital who have been
fully prepared through training and education for the clinical

responsibilities needed to deliver primary health care in the community – mainly health visitors, district nurses, school nurses, practice nurses, community psychiatric nurses, community mental handicap nurses, occupational health nurses, and a range of specialist nurses (NHSME 1993a). The work therefore embraces nursing care, treatment, investigations, support, health promotion, public health and working for health in communities and in alliance with other organisations.

It is our view that entering the debate about names and labels of nursing is to be avoided, because it tends to reflect a version of professional tunnel vision that is pre-eminently concerned with status and results in dividing and therefore weakening the profession as a whole.

It is not surprising if the profession is confused about what terms to use when there are conflicting messages coming from professional leaders. Government policy uses the term primary health care nursing, outlined above, whereas professional policy from the United Kingdom Central Council (UKCC) and the English National Board for nursing and midwifery (ENB) uses the term community health care nursing (UKCC 1994).

We have chosen to use the term primary health care nursing rather than community health care nursing for two main related reasons. Firstly, central policy explicitly states that the drive for change in the NHS should be led by primary health care and general practice. It is therefore consistent to adopt the terminology outlined in *New World, New Opportunities* on primary health care nursing. Critics may argue that taking this route will mean that nursing will be subsumed by the medical model of primary care. We believe that this sort of argument doesn't lead very far, and that nursing should be confident enough and believe in its distinct role to take part, together with other key players namely general practitioners, not only in the delivery of care, but in initiating, leading and evaluating changes that affect nursing and its client groups.

The second related reason is that by using the broad and overarching definition of primary health care outlined above, community health care forms part of it. The community care reforms, and the focus on social care that these imply, gives another meaning to community health care. Therefore confusion potentially arises when the shorthand term community nursing is used.

Community care is the social care provided for people to remain living independently in their own homes or assisted in residential settings. This may be provided by the Local Authority or purchased from other agencies such as the independent sector. Community care is often used loosely as an overarching term meaning all care carried outside of institutions. This is a loose use of the term, because it ignores the health and social care divide; it also overlooks the fact that some community care takes place inside institutions.

There is also terminological confusion over what we call our patients. We have used the terms patient/client somewhat interchangeably, and we have chosen to use the term user in preference to consumer, customer, particularly in the discussion of issues to do with choice and accessibility to the service.

Overview of content

Major and radical change has taken place in the health and social services in the early 1990s. These changes are well known, and include the introduction of contracting and the separation of purchaser and provider functions, as well as the introduction of a health driven strategy with its emphasis on interagency partnerships, and professionals working together to meet targets for health. The central tenets of the reforms are that care provided by the health service should be efficient, effective, responsive, health orientated and appropriate to the user as well as properly evaluated. This means that primary health care nursing is required to focus on: quality assurance; accessibility to services and practitioners; assessment, care management and developing tailored care plans; working collaboratively with other professionals, patients and their carers to ensure continuity; safe, effective, clinical practice; and involving the user at the centre of care. Therefore the major themes of this book are: user-centred services; health promotion; care management and assessment; working together with other agencies, professionals and carers; the shifting balance of care; the meaning of caring and evaluation.

Chapter 1 Policy overview

This chapter introduces and analyses the recent changes in the organisation of the health services, community care and general practice in terms of the influences, challenges and opportunities for nursing. The intention is that it provides the springboard for ideas that are developed and interconnected in different ways in subsequent chapters. The issues covered are consumerism; community care and care management; developments in general practice; health promotion; the shifting balance of care from the secondary to the primary care sector; and the tension between the management-led outcome-driven framework of service development and a professionally-led approach focused on the individual and caring.

Chapter 2 Health-needs profiling

This chapter, written by Christina Victor (Senior Lecturer in Public Health), explores some of the dilemmas inherent in policies that advocate that health care professionals – general practitioners and nurses – should carry out profiles of the health needs of the populations they are caring for. This raises many problems, because as yet the arena of health-needs assessment is an inexact science with many methodological problems. Further, it highlights one of the vital and important challenges for nurses in primary care, whatever their discipline, which is the twin requirement to assess and give care to individuals within the context of assessing and understanding the wider needs of population groups within the community. These demands raise some very difficult questions about the interface of individual practitioners with a wider public health role.

In this chapter the concepts of need, demand and supply are introduced and discussed in terms of their interpretation and application in a complex health service. The sources of health information are explored in terms of their relative usefulness for nursing in primary health care. The wider methodological issues and constraints to the present knowledge in this area are discussed in terms of the implications for primary health care nursing.

Chapter 3 Current issues in assessment

This chapter focuses on methods of individual assessment as a key part of the NHS and community care reforms. Its importance in priority setting, resource allocation, description of case mix and individual care planning is discussed, as well as its relationship with nurse-led approaches to assessment. Assessment is discussed in relation to screening of people aged 75 years and over in general practice, as well as care management and at the interface of primary and secondary care. Examples of good practice are described.

Chapter 4 Interprofessional work

This chapter explores the link between the developing policies for interprofessional collaboration in primary care and the reality in practice. Ideas about teamwork have been batted about for more than 20 years, but there is still remarkably little work that has addressed the issue in relation to patient outcomes. The chapter considers collaboration in terms of the theoretical frameworks, terminology and empirical research. It discusses some examples of interprofessional disputes in primary care, and raises questions of relevance to nursing. Does teamwork signify a loss of the distinctive core of professional expertise and therefore pave the way to deprofessionalisation and multi-skilling? Are personal care and teamwork incompatible? What are the implications for the organisation of primary health care? What is the role of education?

Chapter 5 Quality of care

This chapter considers the tensions for providers and practitioners between the maintenance of quality and the demand for outcome measurement. Quality assurance, including its component parts of standard setting and audit, is analysed in the light of the literature and policy statements. The issue of measuring practice outcomes in primary health care is debated with particular reference to the methodological difficulties in quality assurance. Changes in practice such as nursing development units and health promotion work are used to examine the ways in which practitioners are meeting the challenges of equating quality with effectiveness. User satisfaction is highlighted as a key indicator taking account of different client groups and cultural backgrounds.

Chapter 6 Family carers

The issue of user satisfaction as a measure of quality is developed further in this chapter from the point of view of informal carers. Carer burden is discussed in the light of policies that unequivocally assert that users and indeed carers should have choice and a key role in assessment and care planning. The cornerstones of the reforms, namely service flexibility, accessibility, equality and responsiveness, are explored in relation to the difficulties and experiences of caring. Implications for the practice of nurses in primary health care are addressed, namely multi-agency cooperation in care provision, partnership between informal and formal care and the difficulties of differentiating between meeting the health and social needs of the carer and the dependant.

Chapter 7 New nursing roles in primary health care

Devolution of decision making and the encouragement of the development of services appropriate to the needs of local communities inevitably result in local organisational diversity. These policies, as well as the focus on primary health care as the driving force for change, mean that the roles of nurses in primary health care will change to meet new demands, and new roles will emerge. In the first half of the 1990s the debate has become taut with anxiety as skill mix is confused by grade mix. This is further complicated by arguments on the one hand for deprofessionalisation while on the other there are strong calls, often from managers, for developing the nurse practitioner role. A number of themes are discussed in this chapter: the implications of organisational change such as purchasing; GP fundholders contracting community nursing services; the skill mix and grade mix debate; the tension between deprofessionalisation and the thrust for greater autonomy for nurses, for example, nursing development units, the role of the nurse practitioner and nurse prescribing; the developing role of the practice nurse; specialist nurses. The tension between the contrasting approaches of individualistic care and public health and the importance of education will be addressed throughout.

Chapter 8 Conclusion and future directions

The concluding chapter draws together and integrates the themes of the book. The emphasis on exploration and analysis of the links between policy and practice throughout the book is intended to provide encouragement to readers to challenge and question. Primary health care has no certainties, and as Schon (1992) suggests it is the low ground, the real world with no well-tested methods or clear answers. It is our view that by understanding the influences on development and change in practice, nurses will be enabled to take an active rather than a reactive part in change. At the very least we hope that primary health care nursing may feel better about itself.

Using the book

The book has been jointly conceived, planned and written as a whole. With the exception of the chapter on health-needs profiling by Christina Victor we have both been responsible for different chapters, while contributing to the ideas and the development of others. While the chapters stand alone, the policy overview in Chapter 1 is intended to outline the framework for the integration of themes and ideas throughout the book. This is achieved through cross referencing and by directing the reader to more detailed analysis of particular ideas or points in different sections of the book. During the preparation of this book we identified the need for up-to-date examples of nursing innovations in primary health care. To this end work was commisioned to identify innovatory practice by a review of published material including a range of periodicals, newsletters and selected data bases. This information is integrated within the book, and is also published separately (Ross and Elliott 1995).

Chapter 1
Policy overview

Summary

This overview looks at recent policy trends and current influences on primary health care services and nursing. Radical policy and organisational change in the 1980s and early 1990s are reflected in the shift in the balance of care and the decentralisation of services. This chapter addresses some of the current issues in primary health and community care, examines their origins, and their impact on nursing. These issues include consumerism, community care and care management, general practice, health promotion, the secondary/primary care interface and the shifting balance of care, and the tension between the management and caring cultures of nursing in primary health care.

Pressures for change

The unfolding years of the twentieth century feature major change. There are the demographic changes in the population structure such as the rising number of old people, particularly the very old, the challenge of the major killers – cancers, heart disease and the life-style diseases – the threat of new risks to health such as HIV and AIDS and the re-emergence of old ones such as TB. There are the continuing care needs of people with long-term health problems, and the alienation and social malaise of a society with high unemployment and homelessness. The introduction of new technology and the shifts in political thinking that have challenged the post-war system of welfare require radical new approaches to the organisation and delivery of primary health care services. This chapter looks at the policy and organisational responses to these pressures with a particular focus on the framework of nursing in primary health care.

The context of the reforms

The health and social care reforms of the late 1980s and early 1990s must be understood within the political context and the broader programme of political change in the public sector at that time. Butler (1994) outlines three of the central tenets of the Thatcher government which strongly influenced the development of the reforms. These were: the primacy of a sound economy; the belief that nothing should be done in the public sector that could equally well be done in the private sector; and an underlying assumption that large organisations were inefficient. As Butler (1994) notes, the internal market in the NHS was the product of a political environment that valued wealth above welfare, markets above bureaucracies, and competition above patronage. In addition to health and social services, internal markets and decentralisation of management were introduced into public housing, state education and public road and rail transport.

Theory of internal markets

The term internal market is something of a misnomer, because markets in the classical sense cannot exist in a service sector. Bartlett and Le Grand (1994) identify a number of ways in which the community care market differs from classical economic theory. On the supply side, providers may not be motivated by the need to derive a profit from their work (e.g. voluntary organisations). On the demand side, consumer purchasing power is concentrated in state purchasing agencies – Health and Local Authorities. The term 'quasi-market' is frequently used to emphasise the distinctive context in which economic interactions take place in health care.

The terminology has softened since the early days. For example, purchasing is now more often called commissioning, and increasingly there is a questioning of the principles of imposing a market economy in health and social care. This chapter aims to introduce some of the current issues in health and social care and apply them to nursing in primary care. In particular it will attempt to highlight some of the inherent contradictions between policies which on the one hand promote collaboration between agencies, and on the other value competition; where choice is the political imperative, but where in reality the alternatives are limited.

The internal market in primary health care

This section looks at some of the issues relating to how the internal market works in primary care. Increasingly purchasing in primary health care is being carried out by combined commissioners of Health Authorities and Family Health Services Authorities. The purchasing role is to define the shape and level of local services to meet defined population need and to improve clinical and health-focused outcomes within a service framework of equity, responsibility and efficiency (Bosanquet 1993).

The necessity to develop a needs-led service which takes account of the needs of defined populations requires the involvement of front-line service providers. Historically the information base for planning community nursing services has been limited to crude measures of contact and restricted definitions of task-orientated care. In order to plan services effectively, purchasers need more sophisticated tools, including activity measures of workload and caseload, performance indicators, patient dependency levels, and criteria of clinical outcome. A more detailed discussion of these issues is presented in Chapter 2. All of this is in its infancy, and the challenge for nurses in primary care is not only to describe and articulate their arena of practice as outlined in Box 1.1 and Box 1.2, but to do it in quantifiable terms. Smith *et al.* (1993), in a small exploratory study of the views of providers and purchasers of district nursing, found that two views emerged from purchasers. At one end were the managers who tended to view nurses as biased reporters of clients' needs, supporting a self-regarding and protective professionalism. At the other end of the spectrum were managers who viewed the nurses' involvement in contributing to the purchasing agenda as inevitable and desirable, because of their closeness to the client and their advocacy role.

Box 1.1 Current strengths of nursing services in primary health care

- being available 24 hours a day, 365 days a year
- supporting individuals through major life events
- establishing close relationships with clients
- having knowledge of the local environment and social context
- providing care for sick people in their own homes
- caring for the chronically sick and disabled in their own homes
- taking part in health promotion
- providing a link between agencies and professionals
- working with at risk and vulnerable clients

Choice and the user

Government policy has emphasised the central position of the user in service planning and delivery. This objective is being addressed through several routes. Firstly, the market approach seeks to empower users by giving them a choice between alternatives and the option of exiting from a service if dissatisfied. Secondly, professionals are being urged to involve users in, for example, membership of user participation groups, and assessment and collaborative care planning. Thirdly, the opening up of complaints procedures, and the encouragement of patient satisfaction surveys through the patient charter initiatives, are additional but important ways of increasing the user's voice.

Box 1.2 Future focus of work

- being flexible and responsive
- working collaboratively
- evaluating outcomes
- working for innovation and change
- targeting care to those in need/at risk
- developing partnerships and networks
- developing clinical guidelines
- reviewing quality, client satisfaction and cost

Biggs (1993) points out the inherent inequalities that exist between users and professionals that limit the possibilities of true choice and participation. He identifies these as: different interests, priorities and cultural concerns, as well as effective exclusion from the negotiating arena of contracting. This then raises the question of the extent to which current policy is internally consistent, particularly in the discussion of choice and health care.

One of the ways in which the reforms are intended to provide greater choice and responsiveness to patients is in the implementation of a government strategy of charters for citizens and patients. The general principles of these charters are to ensure that standards, information, choice and complaints systems are promoted, and that helpful, appropriate and sensitive services are provided by receptive professionals at the sharp end of care. Examples of charters in primary care include that introduced for family doctor services, which requires GPs and primary health care teams to set quality standards in practices for care and health promotion, and the recent Community Care Charter designed to monitor the effects of the community care reforms. A patient charter standard on community nursing appointments was also published in late 1994.

The introduction of charters is potentially a device that could be used by nurses to encourage dialogue with user groups to contribute to standard setting and monitoring. One of the difficulties of this is the problem of arriving at sensible definitions of standards and agreeing a methodology for measurement.

Nursing in primary health care has always been patient focused. This comes from the individual one-to-one encounter in the patient's home, the personal and continuous relationship that develops over time through, for example, monitoring child development or caring for patients with continuing care needs. Finally, the nature of work in the community takes staff away from the immediate purview and supervision of nurse management. This creates differences in the role of a nurse working in primary health care compared to that of a counterpart in hospital, particularly in terms of autonomy and responsibility. Paradoxically, despite this close relationship with the patient the position of primary health care nursing is weak and marginal to the acute nursing sector. A parallel with this can be seen in the relationship that general practice has with hospital medicine, which is both resource rich and technologically powerful.

The issue of user-centred care raises the question: how do nurses in primary care know what users want? If these needs can be defined, what forms of response and developments in practice are possible and appropriate? One of the ways in which nurses are responding to users' needs is by setting up carer support groups. The issue of carers is discussed further in Chapter 6. The review of community nursing innovations in the UK, revealed a number of initiatives in the broad area of information giving (Ross and Elliott 1995). This reflects the fact that users and patients increasingly want more information, honesty and involvement in care. The Alloa continence centre was set up by a district nurse in a Scottish health centre to make continence information and advice more freely available. It has a help line, information and appliances available, as well as access to professional advice (Walker 1992). In addition a variety of nurse-led initiatives have resulted in information packs using different presentational media, for example accident prevention (leaflets); preparation of patients for continuing care on discharge (video); prevention of TB (audio tapes); raising awareness and understanding of disability among school children (structured teaching pack for use in a workshop format). Finally, there are other examples of innovative practice, such as a children's bereavement group and the use of 'solution focused therapy', which has been applied in psychiatric nursing to help clients find solutions by identifying areas of personal strength and ability (Queens Nursing Institute 1993).

Community care

The stated aim of the NHS and community care reforms is to create stronger incentives and to increase efficiency and responsiveness by opening up health and social care to competition (DoH 1989c). Since April 1993 social services have had the responsibility for purchasing social care, through care management and assessment. The most clearly defined change was a financial one in that Local Authorities were charged with the responsibility for the finance of all publicly supported long-term care outside the NHS. Social Security funding under income support arrangements has been run down and reallocated through the revenue support grant to Local Authorities. The majority of this reallocation is to purchase packages of care from the independent sector. Thus Local Authorities have become 'enabling' authorities involved with stimulating the independent sector, separating the purchaser and provider functions within social services departments and establishing more effective joint planning towards the objective of seamless care.

There are a number of issues raised by community care, which have been debated in various forums, and by different disciplines (Ross 1990, Lewis 1993, Hunter 1993). These include the conceptual separation between health and social care, joint working (Chapter 4), seamless care, quality care (Chapter 5) and the user view.

Health and social care

The community care reforms are based on the assumption that health and social care can be marketed, delivered, evaluated and funded separately. It is argued that primary health care workers deal in health, whereas social agencies are in the business of social care. This ignores the fact that most health problems are socially defined, and that the majority of people with continuing care needs require assistance from both services and often simultaneously (Hunter and Judge 1988). The community care proposals recommend that a designated care manager should be responsible for the assessment and care plan including the purchase of appropriate and co-ordinated services. In order to provide seamless care across health and social agencies it is essential to consult the user and carer in the development of the plan. The continuing and inevitable tensions at the margins of health and social care have prompted some controversial suggestions that Local Authorities take on a commissioning role for both health and social care (Association of Metropolitan Authorities 1994).

Some of the complexities and difficulties raised by these new policies are further explored in Chapter 3 on assessment and Chapter 4 on interprofessional work.

Care management

Several community care schemes using care management have been piloted and evaluated in Great Britain, most notably in Kent (Challis and Davies 1986), Darlington (Challis *et al.* 1989) and Gateshead (Challis *et al.* 1990). These schemes were targeted on the frail elderly, to reduce admission to institutional care. In Kent and Gateshead the case manager was a social worker performing the core tasks of care management: case finding; screening; assessment; care planning; monitoring; review; and holding control of the resources. The findings indicated increased client morale and quality of care. However, criticisms have focused on the low wages and lack of job security for the helpers, and the lack of any health professional perspective (Bergen 1992). The Darlington project extended the concept, with the care manager being a member of a multi-disciplinary team, with the nursing input intrinsic to the process, and using multi-purpose health care assistants. The findings again showed improvement in morale and a reduction in depression in the clients (Challis *et al.* 1989).

Care management and nursing

The care management proposals identified nurses, among others, as fitting the role of care managers (DoH 1989c). However, the feasibility of this has been questioned, because the concept has been inadequately defined, and has been variously interpreted (Bergen 1994). Bergen surveyed 98 Health Authorities to identify what she defines as case management related activities among community nurses (note that the term case management, imported from the USA, was changed to care management in policy guidance). It is not surprising that the findings showed a variety of roles reported as care management, but the most frequent role was carried out by community psychiatric nurses, and purchasing of services only featured in 13 per cent of cases in contrast to assessment which was undertaken in 97.5 per cent of cases.

There are some practice examples of nurses working in a care manager role, at the purchasing interface with social services, various models of assessment and examples of innovations in interprofessional work. A case study of a district nurse working jointly on assessment with a social worker care manager in two inner-city GP practices showed that although there was increased understanding between GPs, district nurse and social worker of professional roles and different organisational systems, the district nurse's role in care management was limited, because of differences in employment, working structures, information and referral systems and accountability (Ross and Tissier 1994). There are examples of district nurses carrying out joint assessments using a core assessment tool (Korczak 1993), and multi-agency involvement. For example, in South Bedfordshire the Health Authority, Social Services and the Family Health Services Authority have developed an agreed local model of assessment (Pick 1992), and in South Devon a model has been developed to ensure continuous care in discharge policies (Fares 1993).

The implications for nursing of residential and nursing home care

The rapid increase in residential and nursing home care has largely come about through the use of the Social Security budget to fund nursing home places in the late 1980s, the rundown of long-stay facilities in the NHS and probably because of the demographic factors which show a rise in the elderly population, but a reduction in the number of men and women in their middle years able to supply informal care (Harrison 1993). As a consequence, nurses in primary health care are working more in the Local Authority and independent nursing home sector, providing nursing care to patients, teaching, advising and supporting care staff (district nurses), implementing health promotion programmes (health visitors) and carrying out over-75-year-old checks (practice nurses).

Explicit policy guidelines have been laid down for both the NHS and Local Authorities to comply with in respect of the clarification of hospital discharge arrangements, including joint assessments for those people entering residential or nursing home care. This involves nurses, as their advice is often sought on assessment.

All of these changes in practice place demands for more training in, for example, assessment, care management, hospital discharge procedures and purchasing of care packages, so that nurses in primary care can cope with the new challenges in community care.

General practice

The organisation and delivery of care in general practice has undergone tremendous change in the last five years since the introduction of the 1990 GP Contract (DoH 1989d) and GP fundholding. These changes will be discussed in terms of their general consequences for primary care and nursing in particular.

The GP Contract

The GP Contract proposed to provide better choices for the patient, relate remuneration to performance, ensure value for money, and increase accountability (Chisholm 1990). The key changes of the GP Contract include:

- an increased emphasis on capitation payment, which reflected the government's view that the income of general practitioners should be more directly related to the number of registered patients
- some items of service fees have been replaced by target payments for immunisations, cervical cytology, child health surveillance
- additional incentives to run health promotion services, to undertake minor surgery and work in deprived areas
- requirements to provide health checks for certain patients, namely newly registered, those not seen in three years and those aged 75 years and over

Not surprisingly, the demands of the GP Contract have resulted in a rapid increase in practice nurses employed in general practice. This has aroused interest in the role and characteristics of practice nurses and their training needs in relation to health promotion, home visiting and counselling (Ross *et al.* 1994, Atkin *et al.* 1994). Detailed discussion on practice nursing can be found in Chapter 7.

GP fundholding

The NHS reforms included proposals for independent funding for larger group practices with the size of the budget reflecting the relative needs of patients registered in the practice. GP fund-holders are both purchasers and providers.

Glennerster *et al.* (1994) describe the origins of the idea as emanating from Professor Alan Maynard of York University in the early 1980s. Maynard argued that GPs as gatekeepers to services could act as the consumers' informed guides and health service purchasers. This was thought to be the nearest thing to a consumer-led market. These ideas and the American model of Health Maintenance Organisations influenced the Department of Health's proposals.

The original scheme introduced in April 1991 encouraged practices of a certain size (minimum 9,000 patients) and with an adequate management and technical infrastructure to have control of a practice budget to purchase certain non-emergency hospital inpatient care, outpatient care and selected outpatient diagnostic tests. There were also separate budgets for prescribing, and for practice staff salaries. The initial scheme was highly experimental and it has been argued that the rules were invented as it went along (Glennerster *et al.* 1994). Since the initial scheme a number of modifications have been put in place, for example reduction of practice size from 9,000 to 5,000 patients. In addition, fundholders are now allowed to purchase most elective surgery, outpatient attendances and a wider range of community health services including nursing. In some areas general practices have chosen to join together as consortia or multi-funds, which confer similar powers.

Evaluation of a sample of the first wave fundholders by Glennerster *et al.* (1992) showed some positive findings in that fundholders in their study had used the lever of referrals to withdraw from poor or inefficient hospital services, with hospital consultants moving out into surgeries to give outpatients care, and cost savings being made through more accurate prescribing. However, the authors note that these findings are not sufficient, and it is too early to make claims in support of total fundholding.

The issue of fundholders contracting community nursing services has been debated within the nursing profession, but has not received formal evaluation. The District Nursing Association (1993) identified some of the issues for district nurses. These included terms and conditions of employment; professional autonomy and advice; teamwork and partnership; opportunities to influence the contracting process; recognition and priority within the practice of public health and health promotion; community care and care management; professional development; research opportunities; and quality assurance. In health visiting the concerns have focused on the effects contracting would have on the public health role. In a study of views of key players in primary health care in one of the London health regions it was found that health visitors were worried that the contractual obligations of GPs to meet health promotion targets would limit their wider role in health, for example outreach to marginalised groups and those not registered with GPs (Ross and Tissier 1995).

The GP Contract has had far-reaching consequences on the morale, workload and recruitment of new doctors into general practice. These organisational changes have preoccupied the profession and challenged the ethos within general practice of a personal continuing care service to one of managing a business that is concerned with measuring tasks done, recording and remuneration (Morrell 1993). Indeed, Morrell asks whether doctors committed to personal and continuing care will exist in the future or whether they will be 'managers of health shops, health educators for the community or specialoids' (Morrell 1993: 71).

The crisis facing general practice has a parallel in the crisis facing nurses in primary health care. In fact many of the challenges to professional care are the same, but articulated in different ways.

A health strategy for primary health care

The origins and meaning of health promotion

Much has been written about the meaning of health and the scope of health education and, more recently, health promotion. This section considers the policy context and role of health promotion in primary health care, and particularly as regards nursing. One of the most important changes in the philosophy of health care in the 1980s and 1990s has been the increasing recognition that the major challenges lie in preventing life-style diseases. One of the early statements about health was made in 1977 by the World Health Assembly, which resolved that health for all should be achieved by the year 2000.

In 1978 the Alma Ata Declaration made it clear that improving 'basic' living conditions (termed primary health care) was the key to delivery of health for all (World Health Organisation 1978a). Later, in 1984, this was translated into a defined strategy with 38 health targets in the WHO European Region. The 1986 Ottowa Conference (World Health Organisation 1986) produced a Charter for Action which defined five key principles of health promotion:

- building healthy public policy
- creating supportive environments
- strengthening community action
- development of personal skills
- re-orientation of health services

The Ottowa conference was important because it shifted the focus from education for health towards empowerment of individuals and communities. Health education then becomes subsumed within health promotion. Both terms are often used interchangeably.

Although there has been some confusion over the difference between health education and health promotion (Tones 1986), there is some consensus that health education is planned educational intervention individually focused and aimed primarily at the voluntary actions people can take on their own about their own health or the health of others they are looking after. Health promotion, on the other hand, encompasses health education and is aimed at the complementary social and political actions that will facilitate the necessary organisational, economic and other environmental supports for the conversion of individual actions into health enhancement and quality of life. Health promotion thus extends health education to the primary health care focus on social and political action in the expectation that people will be able to lobby for the social changes which provide the opportunities as well as the education to improve their health status (Rawson 1992).

These wide-ranging objectives have been influential in the development of the new public health movement. It has been said that this is characterised by a move away from preoccupation with health protection and immunisation programmes and a return to nineteenth-century public health concerns with structures, environments and ecology (Bunton and MacDonald 1992). Set against this shift in thinking is the existing culture of health policy, which is informed by an approach to health that has emphasised disease, aetiology and clinical diagnosis. Resulting epidemiological explanations of disease patterns and methods of prevention have been criticised for an overemphasis on individuals, in isolation from their social context, and for driving a narrow oversimplified programme that focuses on information giving and advice at the expense of development, enabling and empowerment (Tannahill 1992).

Although government policy remains focused largely on medical problems leading to specific targets such as immunisations (DoH 1989d), important statements have been made about

healthy alliances and the need to work across government departments, industry, business and education as well as the health
sector (DoH 1992). This means that health promotion should
properly take place in a variety of settings, for example in the
workplace and in commercial and leisure organisations, and with
key population groups. This provides nurses in primary care with
tremendous opportunities for taking a public health approach and
working innovatively with previously untargeted population
groups.

Health promotion in primary care

A number of government policy documents have emphasised the
importance of developing health promotion in primary health
care (DHSS 1977), in general practice (DoH 1989d) and in
community nursing (DHSS 1986). This trend has been acceler-
ated by the government policies which emphasise the shift to
primary care and consumerism.

The evidence, however, is that primary health care nursing
and general practice have been slow to realise their full potential
in health promotion. It has been found that nurses have an
inadequate knowledge base for teaching (Syred 1981), avoid
opportunities to talk to patients (Macleod-Clark 1983), and in
the acute setting give priority to 'patient education and information giving' rather than 'encouraging patients and their families
to participate in care' (Latter *et al.* 1992). Turton (1983) has
pointed out the shortcomings in the health education model used
by district nurses, and has provided us with an explanation that
includes conceptual, educational and operational constraints.
Even health visiting, which is the only profession in the NHS
specifically dedicated to prevention and health promotion, has
been criticised for its narrow focus on child development and
protection and the tendency towards giving prescriptive advice
rather than encouraging client participation (Kendall 1993).

The general practitioner has traditionally had an individual and
case-centred approach to prevention, providing 'personal, primary

and continuing medical care to individuals and families . . . he will intervene educationally, preventively and therapeutically to promote his patient's health' (RCGP 1972:1). Although this statement is over 20 years old it remains an important benchmark for general practice. It has been argued, however, that health education in general practice has been slow to develop for a number of reasons including the absence of health education in the medical undergraduate curriculum (Tones 1983), and secondly the pressure from busy workloads, which makes innovation difficult. As Batchelor (1984) points out, the low priority given to prevention is reflected by the item of service payment. It is this principle that was extended to reimburse the health promotion targets of the 1990 GP Contract. This places limitations on the approach and commitment to health promotion; arguably government policy has had an opposite effect by alienating general practice from the priorities of the health strategy, because of overwhelming pressures from their own contractual obligations. It is important that the general practitioner's contribution to health is clarified. This is even more important due to recent changes in health policy: 'General practitioners must translate the hard language of experimental medicine and epidemiology into the warm idiom of daily life . . . the world needs a new kind of doctor' (Tudor Hart 1983: 29).

Practice nurses have taken a major role in the health-promoting activities in general practice, which has become more focused since the introduction of the banding scheme. As well as carrying out health surveillance on registration with the practice, well women, well men and over-75-year-old people, practice nurses are engaged in a wide variety of health clinics, for example coping with asthma, diabetes, hypertension, stress relief, alcohol control and smoking cessation. In addition, they are involved in primary prevention activities such as child immunisation, advice to travellers and family planning.

The exact contribution of the practice nursing role in health promotion has been debated recently following the findings of the Oxcheck study (Imperial Cancer Research Fund Oxcheck

study group 1994). This randomised controlled trial showed
that health checks carried out by practice nurses were ineffective in reducing levels of smoking, but were effective in helping
people to modify their diet and reduce total cholesterol. Since
the improvements were small, however, researchers have now
some evidence to support the view that targeted intervention may
be more useful than blanket health checks. This has been
supported by a larger-scale screening study (British Family Heart
Study 1994).

There are other practice examples of health promotion. Some
have been instigated by district nurses, for example a multi-
disciplinary team taking health messages to the public in a leisure
centre (Thomas 1993a), targeting Asian elders specifically on
heart disease, diabetes and exercise (Edmond 1993), and the
continuing care needs of people with osteo-arthritis (Dargie and
Proctor 1994). In addition there has been some exciting work
developing Health of the Nation priority areas such as sexual
health of teenagers, parenting initiatives, and the streetwise
project in Newcastle upon Tyne.

Shifting balance of care – secondary/primary care interface

Community care has existed as a broad political goal for 30
years. Until the late 1980s, however, there was no concerted
political or professional will to implement the stated objectives.
The change in direction was influenced by the pressure that came
from the reports of the Government's watchdog Audit Commission (1986) and political adviser on health (Griffiths 1988).
In brief, these reports argued that community care lacked a
coherent policy framework, and the delivery of services was fragmented, which endorsed a prevailing culture that 'community
care is a poor relation; everybody's distant relative but nobody's
baby' (Griffiths 1988: iv). The Audit Commission (1992) identified the community health services as the poor relations of the
acute services with inadequately defined service objectives,

resource shortfalls, and boundary problems between agencies. In this report management were criticised for not having developed adequate information systems, outcome measures and quality assurance programmes, nor having encouraged user involvement.

Changing boundaries between hospital and community

Harrison (1993) has identified a number of forces working to change the pattern of service provision in such a way as to reduce the role of the acute hospital, such as:

- Users are seeking greater involvement in service provision, in some areas making their preferences known for patterns of care which reduce hospital use.
- Chronic conditions are becoming more important in terms of caseload than acute illness so that more care has to be provided on a continuing basis.
- New technology is making it possible for GPs to carry out tests in surgeries and health centres and look after more acutely ill patients at home.

These pressures lead to questions about how primary and secondary care should relate to each other and what the division of functions should be as a result of hospital down-sizing and the transfer of capability and skills into the community. This debate is being carried out at all levels, particularly in relation to contracting, and is leading to new patterns of service delivery such as Hospital at Home, outreach, inreach and the development of specialist community nursing services. The increase in day care not only for surgical techniques such as hernia repair, but also for invasive investigations such as cardiac catheterisation, inevitably has consequences for the nature of work being done in the community by the primary health care team.

Closure of the long-term care institutions and the relocation of the frail elderly, mentally ill and people with learning disabilities in alternative community care settings have been implemented throughout the late 1980s and 1990s. Since the NHS reforms there have been rapid changes. In the case of the acute services the level of activity, bed utilisation, and day surgery has risen steadily while the length of stay has fallen (Harrison 1993). The question this raises is whether or not these changes strengthen the role of the acute hospital and further disadvantage community care, because the difficulty of transferring the authority and resources for care from the acute to the primary care sector remains problematic, particularly in an internal market where acute and community trusts are in competition for resources and business. In the light of the above problems as well as the lack of a visionary management in the Community Health Trusts (Audit Commission 1992), perhaps it is not surprising if the major initiatives in the shifting balance of care are coming from the acute sector rather than from the community or from nurses. Arguably there never was a time that potentially offered more exciting opportunities for nurses in primary care to innovate and develop primary care services, as secondary care shifts into the community. There are many constraints to this, however, including marginalisation of nurses from the policy-making arena (McIntosh 1985).

The next section considers how these pressures to improve the interface between the secondary and primary care sectors have influenced developments within nursing in primary health care. The review of innovations carried out by Ross and Elliott (1995) found that there were remarkably few published examples in this area of the shifting balance of care, with the exception of Hospital at Home initiatives (Thomas 1993b) and the use of new techniques such as laser therapy in wound care (James 1994).

Perhaps the fastest area of development is in outreach services. This describes the work of a hospital-based team including nurses in the follow up and support of patients in the community with a view to supporting recovery and avoiding readmission. There are examples of this in an expanding number of specialities ranging from paediatrics to orthopaedics, cardiology and rheumatology. The developments in acute care services at home include providing continuous ambulatory peritoneal dialysis (Simoyi 1993), administering intravenous therapy and home mechanical ventilation (Ferns 1994). These developments raise questions about the appropriate role of the specialist and generalist, the training required for professionals to work in the different context of the community, the need for good communication with other care providers and the importance of avoiding further fragmentation of care.

The hospital/community interface at discharge

Another aspect of the changing balance of care is the consequence of earlier discharges for the primary health care services. It is well known that there are frequent problems at the interface of secondary and primary care, particularly over admission and discharge. There is recent evidence that in spite of the focus on discharge arrangements resulting from the Community Care Act there are still problems in the information provided by hospitals to primary care staff on the discharge of elderly patients (Tierney *et al.* 1994) and the referral to practitioners such as district nurses (Savill and Bartholomew 1994). Earlier discharge has been said to be a factor in rising readmission rates (Henderson *et al.* 1989). Although Victor and Vetter (1985) found no association between length of stay and readmission, their findings suggest that some readmissions were due to a relapse or breakdown of the initial medical condition. In a study of the factors associated with the unplanned readmission of a random sample of elderly patients matched with a control group, Williams and Fitton (1988) estimated that over half the unplanned readmissions were avoidable. There is important preventive work to be done here by nurses in primary health care who are well placed to take a proactive or key worker role, supported by co-ordinated activity from the primary health care team and improved collaboration with hospital and nursing staff and social services.

Changing boundaries in the inner city and London

The problem of delivery of health care in inner cities and the capital is an exemplar of the interface problem between secondary and primary care. It is widely recognised that primary health care in inner London is less well developed than in outer London and beyond. Obstacles and constraints to providing accessible and co-ordinated primary health care have been identified in a number of reports over the last 12 years (Boyle and Smaje 1993). These constraints have to a large extent also inhibited innovation and development in community nursing services (Boyle and Smaje 1993). In recognition of this the government has allocated additional resources known as Tomlinson money to build the primary care capability and infrastructure. Examples of new initiatives include consultant-led clinics in primary care, general practice and nurse practitioner minor illness/injury services in Accident and Emergency Departments, intermediate care facilities modelled on the Lambeth Community Care Centre, and interim care/nurse-led care in acute district general hospitals for patients recovering, but not ready for discharge. While the media and political attention has focused on the particular problems of general practice, there have been a number of initiatives and funding for development projects in nursing, as noted in Box 1.3.

Box 1.3 Initiatives and development projects in nursing

● nurse practitioners in primary care including pharmacies/AE/health centres
● prevention of admission to hospital
● care management
● intensive patient support at home
● intermediate care centres

Evaluation and the use of clinical guidelines in multi-disciplinary audit

One of the key objectives of the health service is the need to establish clinical effectiveness. This comes from an outcome-driven NHS that needs some measure of effectiveness of clinical care to include in contracts. The idea is not new, because over the last decade there has been considerable work on the development of standards/policies and protocols. Recent examples include audit of leg ulcers (McCready 1993), and an assessment of lifting and handling risk (Pilling 1994). These may, however, not necessarily have been based on a thorough and rigorous review of the literature (Humphris 1994), have been agreed in a multi-disciplinary forum, nor have had any contractual implications. There are some examples of audit of multi-disciplinary teamwork, but little in the way of developing consensus on guidelines within a multi-disciplinary context. This is the challenge for primary care, and is a means to connect and make relevant research findings to practice.

The impact of policy change on the morale and caring role of nurses in primary health care

Major and radical change in policy, organisations and practice often leaves individuals feeling helpless, disillusioned and frustrated, particularly when fundamental values and beliefs about the philosophy of care are challenged. Some of the current challenges come from the demand for quantifiable league tables about clients' needs, and for justification of professional help versus cheaper and less-qualified workers. In other words, the 'deprofessionalisation and commodification of a service' (Carrier and Kendall 1995) have implications for deskilling and dilution in standards and quality. It seems that the amalgamation of these pressures and changes has resulted in a crisis of caring, in which nurses feel that there is an increased polarisation between the values of finance and caring, and that the 'special experience of caring', from which they draw meaning, is being diminished (Traynor 1994). Wade's (1993) work on the job satisfaction and morale of community nurses showed that district nurses and health visitors had negative feelings about work, but that practice nurses felt more positive.

At the heart of this crisis is a conflict between a new style management and professional decision making in the health service. Interestingly this polarisation indicates that both opposed groups have the 'needs' of the user as their *raison d'être*. The managers argue that the service must be consumer driven and that resources should be equitably allocated. Professionals believe that their knowledge and understanding of needs brought about by their relationship with patients should be valued.

The consequence of this is that nursing, like general practice, social work and education, is obsessed about the output of care to the detriment of the caring process. Morrell argues that 'in a civilised society the justification for caring may be caring itself' (Morrell 1993: 64). One of the means of access to the therapeutic function of nursing has always been through its more routine tasks. This provides the information and forms the relationship at the heart of the caring role. There is a danger that failure to articulate what this is and failure to demonstrate and evaluate it will lead to a further deskilling of nursing in primary care.

Conclusion

This chapter has discussed the development of current policy and its influence on primary health care nursing. Key themes, such as the response of nursing to the internal market, consumerism, changes in community care and general practice, and the drive for health outcomes and effectiveness, have been introduced and will be picked up again in later chapters of this book. The message coming from this chapter is that standing still is not an option when the ground is shifting underfoot

(Handy 1989). Rather than feeling disempowered by change it is important that practitioners develop the means to question, to debate and to work towards a future that is meaningful and which can be shared.

Chapter 2
Health-needs profiling

Summary

This chapter examines the meaning, underlying assumptions and possible applications of health-needs assessment to populations in primary health care. The concepts and interrelationships between need, demand and supply, as well as the implications for evaluation of health care, are discussed. The various sources of information that can be accessed by nurses in primary health care to carry out health-needs profiles are outlined in terms of their usefulness, advantages and limitations. This includes a discussion of mortality and morbidity measures, population information, deprivation indicators, health surveys and service utilisation data.

Introduction

Resources for both primary and secondary health care are constrained. Consequently at national, district and primary care levels there are lively debates about how the resources available for health care should be spent. This is complemented by an increased awareness of the need to describe, or profile, the characteristics of the populations served by these different agencies and to try to assess the health care needs of particular populations (Stevens and Raferty 1994, Pickin and St Leger 1993). Nurses working at the primary care level, such as health visitors and district nurses, have already contributed to developing neighbourhood or community profiles of the populations they serve. This is a role which will become increasingly more important as the number of fundholding practices increases and as primary care is expected to become more involved in the assessment of health care needs and in the purchasing of health care. The trend towards the development of health-needs assessment and population profiling is also related to the move towards explicit rationalising and prioritisation of health service provision and the examination of the most appropriate mix of skills, both among and within professional groups, required to provide these services. This chapter considers some of the important concepts underlying the activity of health-needs profiling and the sources of data available for nurses and other health care professionals to undertake such activities.

What is health-needs assessment?

In recent years there has been a significant move towards the development of ways of assessing health care needs of populations. The Department of Health recognised in 1988 that 'the provision of health services should be informed by an assessment of health needs' (Pickin and St Leger 1993). The strongest stimulus to the move towards health-needs assessment, however, was the 1989 reform of the National Health Service, and the purchaser/provider split. In order to purchase appropriate health care for their resident populations, commissioning agencies need both to profile, or describe, the characteristics of their populations and to assess their need for health care. Such tasks are often the responsibility of the Public Health Departments. The results of these activities are often made available in the reports of the Director of Public Health and the purchasing plans and intentions of the agencies.

Within primary care there have been parallel developments. The new contract for GPs, introduced in 1990, requires practices to submit an annual report, describing their activities and the population served, to the Family Health Services Authority (FHSA). General practices, especially fundholders, are also having both to profile their population and to assess its need for health care. Those fundholding practices that purchase, or contract, community nursing services will need to establish the level of 'need' among their populations for these services, so that they can purchase the appropriate amount and type of services. Given the emphasis which current policy places upon extending the number of fundholding practices and the areas of care in which fundholders will be given responsibility for purchasing, it seems likely that the needs assessment and population profiling activities of those working in primary care will increase. Indeed the recent Department of Health letter, which proposes a move towards a primary care-led health service, re-emphasises the importance which will be placed upon these activities in primary care (DoH 1994a).

Unlike the situation with health commissioning agencies (currently the purchasing authority for specific geographical areas) those working in primary care have an important conflict of loyalties. General practitioners, health visitors and district nurses are responsible for 'assessing the health care needs of their population' and are also actual providers of care. They must reconcile the competing tensions of being providers of care to individual patients and of implementing the 'rationing' or 'priority setting' decisions resulting from their population or community level health-needs assessment work. For example, health-needs assessment will, almost inevitably, identify previously unmet needs for which resources may not be available, or may recommend that a popular, but ineffective, service be withdrawn. Reviews of the types and grades of staff required to provide the most appropriate patterns of care may generate conflict when it results in changes to the status quo and traditional professional roles. While the full implications of this dual role for primary care and its workforce have not yet been fully worked through, it is clearly an uncomfortable position for nurses and other primary health care workers.

Need, demand and supply of health care

When considering the very broad areas of needs assessment and population profiling, three very important terms – need, demand

and supply – must be distinguished. Need relates to what people would benefit from; demand relates to what people would use in a free health care system, or pay for in a market-based system; and supply describes what is actually provided. Each of these three terms is now considered in more detail.

Need

Need is a word which is very commonly used in everyday conversation. Within a population health context, need has a more specific and technical meaning. For the purpose of this chapter need is defined as the ability of an individual, or population, to benefit from a specific health care intervention (Stevens and Raferty 1994). The need for health care is very much more specific than the need for health. The need for health care is the population's ability to benefit from health care (DoH 1991b) and is contingent upon the existence of services, therapies or interventions to remedy the identified problem.

This chapter is concerned with identifying health needs at a population, not an individual, level. Individual or clinical need takes the patient, or client, as its focus, and need, in this instance, is defined as the 'best' which can be done for a particular patient at a particular time. Traditionally the clinical view of need does not take account of those patients, for example people with depression or hypertension, who do not consult a GP. Neither does a clinical perspective on need take into account the resource implications of treating a particular individual. In this chapter the focus is upon identifying population-based needs. In this context the population under review may be patients from a health centre or the population of a specific locality, or indeed a sub-group of these such as older people or children. This work at the population level requires a change of perspective towards a 'public health'-based world view.

If need is defined in terms of what people would benefit from, this raises the questions of who should define benefit and who should interpret and collect the information. Within both primary

and secondary care, it is important that the term benefit is interpreted widely to include both patients and carers and that the
term should embrace both clinical and non-clinical dimensions.
It is important to remember that need is a dynamic concept.
Services which were 'needed' in the past, such as mass chest
X-ray screening, may outlive their usefulness. The development
of new and worthwhile forms of treatment and interventions will
create new health care needs.

This very broad concept of need may be further sub-divided
into four components (Bradshaw 1972). The basis of the classification is how the health care needs are distinguished. Bradshaw
(1972) distinguishes between the following sorts of need:

- *Normative needs* are those defined or identified by an expert
  or health professional. Within primary care, examples of
  'professionally' defined needs might be identifying health
  problems in a well man clinic and screening surveys of the
  population, such as the over-75-year-old assessments. This
  type of screening may identify health problems which are
  either asymptomatic or which the individual does not identify
  as illness – perhaps putting down the symptoms to old age.
- *Felt needs* are those needs which are identified by individuals,
  for example the desire for more information about giving up
  smoking, advice about hormone replacement, or information
  requested by some pregnant women for a home birth.
- *Expressed needs* are felt needs translated into action, for
  example the demand from pregnant women to use a birthing
  pool, or an older person seeking treatment for arthritis from
  their general practitioner.
- *Comparative needs* are defined by the comparison of health
  care provision received by the population, or a sub-section of
  the population, in one area, with that received elsewhere. If we
  do not know what the optimal pattern of service provision is,
  then simple comparisons between groups and areas may highlight areas of unmet, or overmet, need. The comparative
  approach is especially powerful in the context of capitation

based funding. For example, studies of comparative need may highlight differences between areas in the rates of surgical procedures (Saunders *et al.* 1989) or between men and women as regards access to particular services (Petticrew *et al.* 1993).

Demand

Demand for health care relates to needs translated into action. Demand originates from both patients and primary health care staff. Examples of patient-originated demand would be a smoker who, wishing to quit smoking, consults a GP for advice, or a woman consulting a family planning nurse for contraceptive advice. Doctors and nurses, acting as agents or advocates for the patient, generate demands for health care by referring patients for tests, investigations and second opinions.

The demand for health care services is not necessarily an accurate reflection of the need for services because demands for services are affected by the following:

- *Knowledge of the existence of services* This very simply reflects the fact that an individual cannot use or demand a service if unaware of its existence. For example, smokers cannot attend a primary care-based smoking cessation clinic if they don't know it exists. Inevitably publicity, whether at local or national level, about the existence of a service will increase demands for that service. Similarly doctors and nursing staff who are not up-to-date on treatment and service developments will not be able to give appropriate patient information.
- *The local availability of services* This means that if a service does not exist or is limited in its availability, uptake is affected. For example, health promotion clinics run by nurses in a local health centre that are only available from 9am to 5pm are unlikely to be used by working people. Similarly, working parents may be unable to bring their child for routine developmental checks if such services are only offered during

'working hours'. The existence of a long waiting list for joint replacement may result in some people either not using the service or turning to the private sector. Doctors may be deterred from referring to services which have long waiting lists.

Supply

Supply relates to the availability of particular health care services, but again is not a surrogate for the need for health care. The level of supply of a particular service reflects numerous pressures and constraints, including historical patterns of supply, as well as political, professional and public pressure. In very broad terms health care services, at both primary and secondary care levels, are often regarded as sacrosanct, even when they have long outlived their usefulness. The passion which is inevitably generated when hospital closures are discussed is a good example of this. Additionally, medical innovations such as scanners or routine cholesterol screening are greeted with a demand for implementation even before they have been rigorously evaluated.

The fact that some services are available may well stimulate use, even though they may not be appropriate. In the past social bathing was seen as a district nursing service, but it is increasingly becoming a Local Authority responsibility. In spite of this, in some areas district nurses still get inappropriate referrals for social baths. Doctors may stimulate service use by retaining people in outpatient clinics, recalling patients for a follow-up examination, or keeping people in hospital longer than necessary, because of the need to fill and retain control over beds – sometimes described as tactical bed blocking! District nurses may retain some patients on their caseload after their wounds have healed, because they are not 'quite sure' if everything is back to normal, to prevent recurrence, or perhaps to keep their case numbers up. The importance of supply side factors in generating utilisation of some services should not be underestimated, although its exact impact remains difficult to quantify, and probably varies between different health care services.

The relationship between need, demand and supply

What is the relationship between need, demand and supply? It has already been hinted that the relationship between demand, supply and need is not symmetrical (see Figure 2.1). There are seven main combinations of the concepts of need, demand and supply. These may be broadly divided into those where there is a need but no demand or supply, those where there is supply but no demand or need and those where there is demand but no need or supply. Then there are varying combinations. The different combinations and some examples are outlined on p. 34:

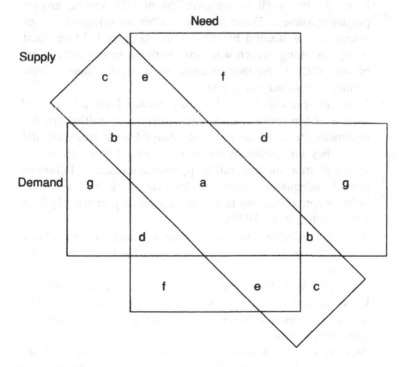

Figure 2.1 The interrelation between need, demand and supply
Source: After Stevens and Raferty 1994

a. *Interventions or services needed, demanded and supplied* – identifies areas of both primary and secondary health care provision where there is a direct overlap between these three factors and identifies a variety of aspects of care including providing home births, childhood immunisation, cervical cancer screening, or domiciliary care of the terminally ill.

b. *Some services will be demanded and supplied but are not needed* – e.g. demands from 'the worried well' for HIV testing following publicity about HIV.

c. *Some services may be provided but not needed or demanded* – e.g. 'wholesale' assessment or screening of particular population groups, such as the over-75s or HIV testing among pregnant women. These may be neither an effective use of resources nor wanted by the clients concerned. Mass chest X-ray screening, which was very pertinent in the early years of the NHS, is another example of a service that is now neither demanded nor needed.

d. *Some services will be needed and demanded but not supplied* – such as hip replacements where there is a waiting list for treatment. Patients may not be discharged home from hospital when they are medically fit for discharge if there are insufficient district nursing staff to provide aftercare. A failure to provide adequate amounts of long-stay care may result in older people remaining in hospital for an inappropriately long time (Victor *et al.* 1993).

e. *Services needed and supplied but not demanded by consumers* – such as campaigns to promote physical activity among the inactive.

f. *Services which are needed but not demanded or supplied* – known as unmet need (see below), such as treatment for undiagnosed illness like hypertension or dementia, or rehabilition following a stroke or a heart attack.

g. *Services may be demanded by individuals or groups but are neither needed nor supplied* – e.g. patients with terminal illnesses, for whom all effective interventions have been provided, but who may still demand help even though no further help is possible.

Unmet need

Figure 2.1 highlights in particular the issue of unmet need. This is defined by sector f in the diagram, which illustrates that for many conditions there may be extensive needs existing within the community which are neither identified by primary health care workers nor provided for. This is well illustrated by surveys of elderly people living in the community that inevitably and universally identify extensive amounts of previously unrecorded illness or morbidity (Williamson *et al.* 1964).

Unmet need for health care is probably extensive and it is well recognised that only the 'tip of the iceberg' of illness is actually translated into the active seeking of medical services by patients (Hart 1985). For a variety of reasons, including the patients' perception of their own health status, for example putting down symptoms to 'old age' rather than illness, or because of the attitudes of family and friends or the accessibility and availability of health care services, only a minority of the total pool of illness within the community actually reaches the health professionals. Figure 2.1 also indicates that, in some cases, services which are no longer required may continue to be provided and demands for inappropriate services may be made. The complexity of the relationship between these different concepts exhorts us to look critically at the health care system and provision overall.

Evaluation of health care

The whole underpinning of needs assessment is the provision to patients of services, therapies or interventions which are of proven benefit. This then raises the problem of which interventions are beneficial and how this is determined. Although there is much more interest now being expressed in the importance of evaluation in health care (St Leger *et al.* 1992), it remains unfortunate that remarkably few health services have been evaluated. It has been estimated that only 20 per cent of health service interventions have been evaluated and found to be of proven benefit (Hoare 1992). This section raises some of the issues and questions concerning evaluation that are pertinent to the development of primary care based needs assessment and profiling.

In attempting to evaluate any health care intervention Maxwell (1984) suggests that six issues need to be addressed:

- *Evaluation* Within this context evaluation relates to the 'scientific' assessment, in as rigorous a way possible, of the extent to which health services, or their constituent parts, such as diagnostic tests, achieve their stated goals. For example, does an anti-smoking programme result in people quitting smoking, and do HIV awareness campaigns increase the use of condoms?
- *Effectiveness* This investigates the most basic aspect of the outcome, or result, of a particular intervention. Outcome resulting from health care interventions is usually described in terms of survival, recovery, restoration to full functioning and quality of life. For example, what is the outcome of offering dialysis to older people with kidney disease, and what is the outcome for older people with arthritis of introducing a structured care package?
- *Efficiency* This is an economically based measure and describes the relationship between the resources put in and the outputs from a service. This is a very difficult concept to measure in health care-based studies. It is worth noting, however, that services can be both efficient but also ineffective. For example, a trial of multi-phasic screening in general practice identified a significant amount of previously unreported morbidity in the screened population (South East London Screening Group 1977). Most of these problems, however, were of a minor nature and at the end of the study

there was no difference in the outcome between the screened group and a control group. This is an example of a very efficient but ultimately ineffective service.

- *Acceptability* This is a neglected but important concept in both needs assessment work and evaluation studies, and one which should be at the forefront of every health professional's consciousness. If the health service is unacceptable to potential users, then, regardless of its effectiveness or level of efficiency, it will not be used. This dimension of evaluation deals with the way in which a treatment or service is delivered and is largely concerned with issues of quality. Is it delivered humanely? What do the patients think of the service? Would you be happy for one of your family to be cared for in this way? Issues such as providing culturally appropriate care fall within the broad concept of acceptability. This is a difficult but vital aspect of evaluation to measure.

- *Appropriateness* This relates to the selection of the 'most appropriate' method of treatment or service delivery for a particular health care problem or client group. An intervention can be appropriate only when certain criteria are met. The intervention should be performed only if appropriate and adequate resources are available and if it is undertaken in a way that is acceptable to the patient. For example, procedures that can be performed using keyhole surgery, and which therefore have a short recovery time, may be more appropriate for patients who are working. Conversely, 'day' surgery may be less appropriate for older people, who may not have anyone to look after them at home when they are discharged.

- *Accessibility* This relates to the access to services and considers whether individuals get the treatment that they need. Again this is a multi-faceted concept as it relates to the barriers which may or may not exist to people using services, such as distance to services, transport, access for the disabled, and the operation and opening hours of clinics and other health care facilities. Other aspects of the concept of accessibility include access to the decision making process and access to information about health matters in general and the services offered. As for the various aspects of access, there are issues regarding the right of access, the ease of access and the cost of access which require consideration.

Sources of information

Whatever type of needs assessment or population profiling activity the primary care worker is involved in there is an obvious and very fundamental need for relevant and appropriate information. This section considers the types of information of interest to those undertaking such projects. Within a single chapter it is not possible to offer a detailed review and critique of sources of data. Therefore this discussion concentrates upon the most widely available and routinely used health and health-related data. Before considering the merits and drawbacks of these data sources, it is first necessary to describe some of the key terms used in the presentation of such data.

Describing health and disease in populations

Two key concepts in describing health and disease in populations are incidence and prevalence. When attempting to develop community profiles and locally based needs assessment, primary health care staff will need to be familiar with both these concepts and their methods of calculation.

Incidence may be defined as the number of new cases of a specific disease occurring within a defined population during a given time period (see Box 2.1). Although typically used to describe the number of new cases of a disease, it is easy to see that the notion of incidence has a wider applicability, as it could also be used to describe the number of new smokers generated annually. As such, the calculation of incidence rates can be a very informative activity for primary care workers seeking to understand the population which they are serving.

Box 2.1 Definition and calculation of incidence and prevalence rates

1) Incidence

- $$\frac{\text{number of new cases of dementia in 12 months}}{\text{Total population aged 65+}} \times 1,000$$

$$= \frac{40}{6,000} \times 1,000 = 6.6 \text{ per } 1,000 \text{ aged } 65+$$

2) Prevalence

- $$\frac{\text{total cases of dementia}}{\text{total population aged 65+}} \times 1,000$$

$$= \frac{600}{6,000} \times 1,000 = 10 \text{ per } 1,000 \text{ population aged } 65+$$

Prevalence records the number of cases of a specific disease (e.g. dementia) in a defined population at a specific point in time (see Box 2.1). Although incidence and prevalence rates are usually used to measure disease, they may also be used to describe aspects of life-style relevant to the development of profiles in primary care. For example, we may calculate the number of new smokers (incidence rate) as well as the prevalence of smoking in particular areas or populations.

It will be seen later in this chapter that there is a variety of readily available health indicators and these may be used to build up a profile of the health of the population served by the primary health care team. National data may also be applied to local populations in order to describe the extent of particular problems. For example, Table 2.1 illustrates how national data about the prevalence of dementia have been used to estimate the number of people with this disease in a hypothetical general practice. Using a similar methodology it would be possible to estimate the number of heavy drinkers or smokers in a local population, or the number of stroke patients, that the practice might expect to see over a given period.

Table 2.1 Application of national prevalence data for dementia to a practice population

Estimated prevalence of dementia (%)	Age group	Total population in practice	Estimated cases of dementia
0.5	60–64	1000	5
1.1	65–69	900	10
3.9	70–74	800	31
6.7	75–79	600	40
13.5	80–84	400	54
22.8	85–89	200	46
34.1	90+	100	34

Incidence rates are extremely useful measures for those concerned with health planning or needs assessment, as they indicate how many new cases of a disease, or particular form of behaviour such as smoking, might be expected over a particular time period, e.g. a year. Changes in incidence rates show whether or not a particular disease or problem is increasing or decreasing in size and also reflect the changing size of the 'population at risk' of particular health problems. Incidence rates form a useful measure for the evaluation of the effectiveness of many primary care-based activities. It may be inferred that decreasing incidence rates indicate the success of health promotion or disease prevention strategies or therapeutic interventions.

Both the notions of incidence and prevalence are problematic, because they are based upon the assumption that we may unambiguously classify the population or individuals into two distinct and discrete groups – those with the disease or problem behaviour and those without. For many conditions or aspects of behaviour which are of interest to those in primary care this is problematic because there are rarely situations in which individuals may be unambiguously described as having or lacking the condition or behaviour under review. This is particularly problematic for chronic conditions such as dementia where there is a continuum ranging from no impairment to total impairment (see Figure 2.2).

Similar problems apply if we are looking at the prevalence, or incidence, of hypertension within primary care. How high does blood pressure have to be before it is unambiguously classified as 'high'? How many 'high' readings must an individual have in order to be defined as having high blood pressure? Even dividing a population into smokers and non-smokers is not as simple as it might seem at the outset. How are ex-smokers classified? What about pipe smokers? How do you classify those who smoke only monthly? Such questions must be answered when seeking to come up with a smoking-based classification of the population.

Deciding at which point along the continuum illustrated in Figure 2.2 dementia or hypertension are defined (known as the case-definition threshold) will greatly influence the size of the

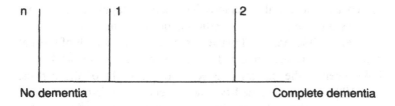

Figure 2.2 Case definition threshold and the disease continuum

identified problem. As Figure 2.2 shows, there would be a much
smaller number of people within the population defined as having
dementia if the threshold were at point 2 instead of point 1. Such
problems are especially acute when we attempt to define the
extent of certain behaviours in our population, such as dietary
habits, or the number of units of alcohol it is 'safe' to consume
on a regular basis, or how much exercise individuals should take.

Population information

The most basic pieces of information required for any form of
needs assessment or population profiling are the size and characteristics of the population under review. Accurate population
data are fundamental to the development of sound needs assessment as these both indicate the size of particular client groups
which are of interest (e.g. older people) and provide the denominators for the calculation of both incidence and prevalence rates
described earlier. The population census is the source of our most
accurate and detailed population data.

In England and Wales the first complete census was undertaken
in 1801. Since then there has been a full census every 10 years,
with the exception of 1941. The last population census took place
in 1991. The aim of the census is to provide a full count of the
population and to collect data about the main characteristics of
the population, such as age and sex structure. The census is
conducted, analysed and disseminated by a government department, the Office of Population Censuses and Surveys (OPCS).

The precise information that is collected varies from census
to census, but usually includes basic demographic information,
such as age, sex, marital condition, place of birth, occupation,
number of children, usual place of residence and length of present
residence. Data are collected about every person in the household, even if the person is absent on the night of the census.
The 1991 census included two new pieces of information never
previously collected, namely self-defined ethnic origin and a
question about chronic health problems. In addition, the head of

the household has to provide details of the residence, including its type, tenure, accommodation and facilities. Direct measures of income or 'social position' are not explicitly collected. Data about car ownership, an indirect measure of social group, is collected, however. Information about the number of adults in employment, and those unemployed, is collected as are details about the types of jobs held by the employed and retired. It is these data which form the basis of the social class classification data provided by the census. All the information relating to individuals is confidential, even within government departments.

Census information is made available in a variety of different formats. Published tables provide information about specific topics, such as pensioners and ethnic minorities, or about specific geographical areas, for example Great Britain, regions and parishes. Only very limited amounts of the wide spectrum of potential data are, however, routinely published. Raw data on computer disks for analysis are also provided which enable local workers to build up more detailed profiles of their local areas. Typically, public health departments provide such detailed analyses in the public health report.

The way in which census data are provided can, however, be problematic for those working in primary care as their population catchment rarely corresponds to administrative areas for which census data are routinely made available (Young and Haynes 1993). Consequently, to develop accurate profiles, groups of enumeration districts may need to be aggregated and data produced for these 'designer' areas. This activity is a very specialist type of activity and is very time consuming. Consequently, population profiles for primary care may only be approximations to the 'true' area served, because of difficulties in defining accurately the spatial area served by a practice and because such areas are not coterminus with other health and social services administrative areas.

Although it is a legal requirement that people should complete census forms, the census does not manage to enumerate everybody. It is estimated that, in 1991, 2 per cent of the population were not included in the census. This is important because this percentage is not equally distributed across the population. Specific groups or geographical areas are systematically under-represented by the census. This means that for these areas or groups census data are inherently biased. For example, in Kensington, Chelsea and Westminster HCA it is estimated that 7 per cent of households did not have their census forms collected, or did not complete their forms. The highest rates of non-completion were among men, those aged 16–29 and members of minority groups (Victor and Lamping 1994). Nationally it has been estimated that 1 million people were missed by the census, especially the groups previously described and those aged 85 and over. Furthermore, homeless people, refugees or other marginal groups may be excluded from the census. Consequently, the health needs of particular populations may be underrecorded.

Furthermore, because the census takes place only every decade, the information which is routinely used by those under-taking needs assessment work can become out of date. While there are estimates of the way in which the size and age–sex composition of the population is changing between censuses, there are no ways of routinely reviewing the accuracy of data about the social characteristics of the population. For instance, revised estimates of the size and demographic composition of, for example, minority communities are not made available.

For planning purposes it is often essential to have some idea of the likely size and composition of the population in years to come. The essential difference between population estimates and population projections is that an *estimate* is based on knowledge of the births, deaths and migration that have happened, and a *projection* is based upon what is thought likely to happen. Therefore assumptions are made about trends in mortality, birth rates and migration. These projections are likely to be less reliable the further forward they are made, because the assumption of birth and death rates is likely to be increasingly inaccurate. Like population estimates, population projections are not made for small areas, such as wards or the areas served by clinics or health centres, because of statistical unreliability. The combination of these factors means that health professionals working in small localities or areas may often be basing their activities on inaccurate population data. This limitation should be noted when presenting population profiles based upon out-of-date census data. In many situations, however, there are no alternative sources of data and the primary care worker has to use what is available.

Alternative sources of population-based data

Given the problems which primary care staff may experience in using census data in developing needs assessment and population profiles, the question arises as to whether or not there are any alternative sources of information available. Potential sources of data are the practice lists kept by each primary care team. If computerised in an appropriate format these could provide a breakdown of the age and sex composition of patients registered with the practice. In the past, however, these data have been shown to be highly inaccurate, because patients who have left the practice have not been removed from the list. This is known as list inflation and can be up to 30 per cent in some inner-city districts. Similarly, population estimates or denominators derived from clinic registers are notoriously inaccurate, because of the failure to keep registers up to date and to remove cases which have been closed.

Jefferies *et al.* (1991) examined the apparently low rates of immunisation among children in an inner-London Health Authority. Out of a cohort of 1,485 children identified from clinic records as being eligible for the DPT immunisation, 462 were recorded as non-immunised. Detailed research revealed that of this 462, 195 were in fact fully immunised and 176 children were erroneously listed as they had left the area. Similarly, Beardow *et al.* (1989) reported that of 687 women invited by the Family Health Services Authority for cervical screening, 477 were either not eligible or no longer resident at the address. These are two issues which any primary care needs assessment might include. Although the levels of inaccuracy in the GP and child health computer system were very large in these studies, they do serve to highlight the problems of using practice and routine data systems to provide population data.

Measures of deprivation

In addition to using individual census variables, such as the number of those aged 65, or the percentage living alone, considerable interest has been expressed in using combinations of variables to generate indices of deprivation. The rationale for developing such measures is that those who experience material and social deprivation experience the worst health and have the greatest need for health care. Scores such as these are increasingly being used in allocation of health service funding, For example, primary care practices with 'high' Jarman (1983) deprivation scores receive additional funding to compensate them for the additional health needs these impose. While it is unlikely that primary care staff would be involved in calculating such scores (this is usually done by regions or by academic departments with the necessary expertise) they would be part of any needs assessment or population profile. As such it is important that nurses know why such scores developed and what the main limitations of such measures are.

There are three widely used measures of deprivation: the Townsend *et al.* (1988), Carstairs and Morris (1989) and Jarman (1983) scores. The variables included in the calculation of these measures are shown in Box 2.2. A range of criticisms has been levelled at these composite deprivation measures, especially the increasing role they play in resource allocation and the way in which such indices take on a life of their own. The inclusion of ethnicity data in the Jarman index has been a source of contention as it is argued that this biases the index in favour of London (Talbot 1991). Furthermore, the index was originally devised to measure general practitioner workloads, not deprivation. There are further technical criticisms of the index to do with methods of computation and the spatial units upon which the index is calculated.

Mortality

It remains a paradox of health-needs assessment work that our most reliable source of data about the health of the population relates to data about deaths. Information about the number and causes of deaths is available for the UK and its constituent areas.

Box 2.2 Variables included in major deprivation indices

1) Townsend *et al.* 1988 index

- overcrowding
- lack car
- non owner occupation
- unemployment

2) Carstairs and Morris 1989 index

- overcrowding
- lack car
- male unemployment
- low social class

3) Jarman 1983 index

- elderly living alone
- children under 5
- lone parents
- unskilled workers
- unemployed
- overcrowding
- changed address
- ethnic minorities

Registration of death is compulsory and a doctor is required to certify the cause of death. The information which is recorded is as follows:

- date and place of death
- name of deceased
- sex of deceased
- place of birth
- date of birth
- occupation
- usual address

The medical practitioner certifying the death is required to record the 'immediate' cause of death and then any underlying disease or condition which led to the death. The precision with which cause of death is identified varies considerably and is generally much less accurate for older people than for those in younger age groups. It is almost inevitable that some causes of death which carry a considerable social stigma, such as AIDS, are underreported. Consequently it would be difficult for a general practitioner to examine mortality from AIDS within the practice, because it is likely that the 'true' number of AIDS deaths may be larger than those actually ascribed to AIDS. Similarly, a district nurse wishing to examine the number of deaths resulting from hypothermia will inevitably underestimate the problem, because of the under-recording of deaths from this cause.

Death registration data are collated and analysed by the Office of Population Censuses and Surveys (OPCS). Mortality statistics are presented in a variety of forms, including the total numbers of deaths, geographical variations, causes of death and mortality rates. Data are published routinely for a variety of geographical areas such as counties or Health Authority districts. Routine data are not, however, usually made available for very small areas such as wards. Consequently, to present a profile of the major causes of mortality within a partic-ular community would probably involve the collation and analysis of individual death certificates – a long and time-consuming occupation.

The paucity of true morbidity measures has led many health service planners, and those responsible for resource allocation, to use mortality statistics because of their availability. This is justified by the view that, on the whole, when mortality is high then so is morbidity. While current patterns of mortality may identify the areas or groups with poor health, they may, however, give a very poor picture of the present health risks of living in a particular community. For example, data about the extent of mental health problems in the community are not well covered by mortality data, because mental illness is not an important cause of death, but is the cause of considerable mental ill health within the population. Similarly, a health-needs assessment for those aged 65 and over based upon mortality data would identify heart disease, cancer and respiratory disease as the main health problems, while a morbidity-based analysis would highlight the issue of osteo-arthritis and accidents (Victor 1991).

If a mortality profile is to be developed for a clinic or practice, it is rarely sufficient simply to count up the number of deaths over a given period, usually 12 months. The total number of deaths gives only a partial view of the patterns of mortality within any given population. It is usually necessary to go on to calculate a variety of different mortality rates (see Box 2.3). Data from census and mortality information are brought together to express the number of deaths as a percentage of the population 'at risk'. The arithmetic involved in calculating such rates is very straightforward (see Box 2.3). As discussed in an earlier section, however, problems can be experienced in getting hold of the census data and with the rapid 'outdating' of the population denominators as we move away from the census year.

Morbidity measures

Morbidity statistics are concerned with the amount and types of illness that occur within the population. Most routinely collected

Box 2.3 Calculation of mortality rates

A) Crude death rate

$$\frac{\text{total deaths in population (numerator)} \times 1,000}{\text{total population (denominator)}}$$

B) Age specific death rate

$$\frac{\text{deaths in women aged 65–74} \times 10,000}{\text{total women aged 65–74}}$$

C) Age and cause specific death rate

$$\frac{\text{deaths from breast cancer for women aged 65–74} \times 100,000}{\text{women aged 65–74}}$$

D) Perinatal mortality rate

$$\frac{\text{stillbirths and deaths within 7 days of birth} \times 1,000}{\text{total live and still births}}$$

E) Infant mortality rate

$$\frac{\text{deaths of live born children within 12 months of birth} \times 1,000}{\text{total live births}}$$

morbidity data suffer from serious shortcomings, partly because of the variable nature and imprecise diagnosis of many illnesses and partly because of inadequacies in the information systems.

The main routinely available morbidity statistics are as follows:

- statutory notifications of infectious diseases
- notification of episodes of sexually transmitted diseases
- notification of 'prescribed' and other industrial diseases and accidents

- notification of congenital malformations
- registration of handicapped persons
- cancer registration

As this list indicates, these data are only a very limited conceptu-
alisation of 'health' and are very dependent upon accurate
identification and notification by medical practitioners. This probably means that for some conditions the notifications rep-resent
only a minority of the actual, or 'true', numbers of cases.
Furthermore, not all these data relate to individuals – some, like
the sexually transmitted diseases notifications, relate to clinic
attendances NOT to individuals. Such data are almost never available for the areas served by a primary health care centre or clinic.

Surveys of health status

Limited data about the overall health of the national population
are available from several sources. The 1991 census included a
question about the number of individuals within households with
'long-term limiting illness'. This is a very broad indicator of the
prevalence of chronic health problems within the population. At
both local and national level it correlates very well with data
about mortality. As these data are available for small areas this
measure may be a good way of identifying particular localities
or districts which are experiencing health problems.

The General Household Survey (GHS), an annual social survey
undertaken by OPCS, also collects data about the prevalence of
both acute and chronic health problems. Because of sampling
issues, however, data are not available for areas smaller than health
or statistical regions. Of more use to those interested in health
promotion are the data collected by the GHS about smoking habits,
alcohol consumption and exercise. Again, however, such data are
not available for areas smaller than regions. Also the GHS included
within its study population only those adults resident in the community. Excluded from the study are those resident in institutions,
such as nursing and residential homes, prisons, etc. This may limit

the usefulness of the data that the survey may provide to those working in primary care.

OPCS also sponsor a variety of ad hoc surveys looking at health issues. For example, they undertook a survey of the prevalence of disability within the population (Martin *et al.* 1988) and in 1985 they undertook a special survey of carers as part of the GHS (Green 1988). The ad hoc surveys are centred upon a specific topic and often provide data about smaller areas than the GHS. They do not, however, always collect the precise data a researcher ideally would like. Again they are often a useful source of broad prevalence rates, which can then be applied to the particular primary care context and can provide nursing staff with a broad indication of the scale of different problems within the communities which they serve.

Service utilisation data

Service utilisation is another, but less satisfactory, measure of morbidity. The majority of these data derive from administrative returns collected by the NHS and have only limited use in health-needs assessment. In theory at least, NHS data have the strengths of being relatively cheap, comprehensive and consistent. Korner data for inpatient episodes are extensive and include a wealth of data concerning the hospital stay. These data are collated centrally and eventually published, but rarely for administrative areas smaller than regions. Routinely published information is available on completed consultant episodes, waiting times for admission and first and all admissions to mental hospitals. Within primary care, nurses working in community settings complete Korner returns. These detail the number of contacts seen, their age, gender and the broad reason for the contact, as well as details of the date the contact took place and possibly place of contact. The main problems with routine NHS data sources relate to the completeness and accuracy of the data (McKee 1993).

The majority of the routine activity data which are readily available are of little use to those working in primary care as they are focused upon the secondary care sector. With the notable exception of Korner data there is a paucity of data available describing the activity of primary care workers. The Family Health Services Authority (FHSA) takes data from the practices within its area and produces a variety of indices including immunisation and cervical smear rates. As we saw earlier, however, data from these sources are notoriously inaccurate because of errors in the population denominators used.

Overall routine administrative data collected by the various branches of the NHS are of limited use because of:

1. the incomplete nature of the data, e.g. failure to record important pieces of data such as diagnosis
2. errors in the accuracy of the information which is recorded, e.g. diagnosis being miscoded or date of discharge inaccurately recorded
3. the inaccessibility of much of the data

Conclusion

Health-needs assessment and population profiling are activities of considerable importance at both local and national level. The recent health strategy, *Health of the Nation*, has served to highlight how little readily available data are available about the health and health habits of our population. The establishment of specific targets within this strategy will probably serve as an impetus to improve the range and quality of the available data. For all but a few topics, however, we have to continue to adapt existing data to fit the purposes for which we wish to use it. Within primary care the development of computerisation offers one way of improving our knowledge of the health of the population served and its need for health care interventions. Although the majority of general practices are now computerised, many systems are currently used for prescribing. Few systems hold patient-based information. By combining the age and sex register with selected information, such as details of smoking or the presence of a chronic illness, however, practices can build more accurate profiles of the populations they serve. Computerisation of details about prescribing and hospital referrals will enable the primary care workers to look at how they are managing the health care problems of their population and to consider how effective those treatment regimes are. Such developments would then enable primary care to develop services which are effective, appropriate and responsive.

Chapter 3
Current issues in assessment

Summary

The aim of this chapter is to explore the issue of individual assessment within the rapidly changing policy context of primary health and community care. This builds on the previous chapter, which looked at the role of population-needs assessment at the public health end of the continuum. Assessment is advocated as a cornerstone of the NHS and community care reforms. Nurses in primary care have always carried out some form of patient assessment, but today it is increasingly important not just for individual care planning, but also for priority setting, resource allocation and description of case mix. The purpose of this chapter is to discuss assessment within the context of policy changes introduced by the community care legislation and the GP Contract. In addition, it discusses some recent work in the development of standardised measures of assessment. While the principles of assessment are largely generalisable, particular examples from care of the elderly are given.

Assessment and the policy context

The new requirements of nurses and other health providers to develop and refine assessment strategies have to be understood within the context of recent changes in policy (see Chapter 1). These changes have emphasised the central importance of assessment in the conceptual and operational split between the provider and purchaser roles. The community care legislation, care management and market pressures on the delivery of care demand that effective mechanisms for assessment are in place in order to target interventions, predict outcomes and plan flexible packages of care that reflect user and carer choice and ensure quality care. Despite the rhetoric, however, there are many complicated issues at the heart of the assessment debate, and these are listed in Box 3.1.

Box 3.1 Key policy issues in assessment

- the meaning of assessment
- the fragmented organisational and value frameworks in primary health and community care within which assessment must be carried out
- definitions of health and social need
- the lack of suitable and properly validated methods of assessing need
- joint working in assessment

The meaning of assessment and conceptual issues

Assessment is a key part of professional practice, and the first stage of the nursing or health visiting process. The language of assessment tends to be profession specific. While doctors may talk about scientific method and the diagnostic process, nurses use the term assessment to include the gathering of data from patients and carers through observation, interviewing and listening to cues. The concept of problem solving is common to both medicine and nursing, and comprises a process of deductive and inductive reasoning. In other words, the professional assessor makes connections between data derived from a variety of sources and in a variety of ways, based on scientific knowledge, 'reflection in action and on action' (Schon 1992), which lead to a hypothesis that can then be tested, validated and evaluated.

There are many important principles that should guide assessment. The importance and value attached to these principles depend on the individual's framework or philosophy of practice. It is these issues that are often debated, not only within professional groups but across professional boundaries. Some examples are given below:

- the continuous process of assessment and review, particularly in continuing care
- assessment of carers' needs alongside the patient
- patient-centred rather than professionally defined assessment
- access to information from other professionals and agencies and the implications for confidentiality
- the appropriate balance of multi-disciplinary and specialist assessment
- acknowledgement of the importance of intuitive assessment and reflective practice
- the link between assessment, outcomes and evaluation

Thus the nature of assessment is complex. The above list raises some selected issues, but the key point concerns the purpose of the assessment and who is going to benefit. In other words, who is setting the agenda? There may be assumptions made about disability, dependency, need and expectations of care that lead to conflict between the patient and the assessor. There is a danger that many professional assessments are made on the basis of one encounter, which may lead to a snapshot assessment and labelling. Most importantly, the approach should be patient centred, beginning from the patients' concerns, rather than defined by a particular professional approach and a checklist of questions.

This chapter focuses on some of the issues underlying assessment with which nurses and other professional groups in primary health and community care are currently struggling in their interpretation and implemention of the new policy changes. As the demands for primary health care become ever more complex, and the need for professionals to work together becomes more urgent, clarification of the terms and language used by different professional groups is needed in order to work towards a common and shared language in assessment.

The use of terms

There is a profusion of different terms that describe different approaches or aspects of assessment. These are often used loosely, can be confusing and need defining.

Functional assessment is the identification of baseline information of health and social need from which a plan of care is constructed (Dickinson and Young 1990). It may also be used as a measure of case-mix severity and as an instrument to determine the allocation of resources or to monitor change over time.

Screening is the early identification of treatable disease (McKeown 1968). It seeks to diagnose the symptomatic stage of disease in a defined population using a validated test, so that treatment or social support can be initiated to improve the quality of life and reduce the functional handicap produced by that disease. The test should be appealing, feasible and effective. This means that not only should the problem be clearly defined, but the target population, stage of detection, tests and treatment on offer should be specified. The term screening is often inappropriately applied to the assessment of people over 75 years in general practice – otherwise known as the health check.

The health check is the term introduced by the 1990 GP Contract. The central purpose of the health check is to identify problems at an early stage so that they can be alleviated or at least contained (Williams 1992).

Case finding is initiated by a health professional to detect hidden problems either during routine surgery work or, for example, as part of a health visitor's preventive work (Davies 1990). This is sometimes known as opportunistic prevention.

Nursing diagnosis is a tentative statement or hypothesis regarding a health problem or issue which is amenable to nursing intervention (McMurray 1993). The concept has gained currency in the United States, and according to Mason and Webb (1993) needs to be considered in terms of its applicability in the UK. In the past, nurses have avoided the term diagnosis, because of its connotations with the medical model of care. The introduction of nurse prescribing and the emergence of the nurse practitioner role, however, mean that the place of nursing diagnosis along-side assessment, data collection and problem solving needs to be examined.

Nursing assessment in primary care

Nurses in primary care have traditionally used a number of different assessment models, for example the problem-orientated nursing process. Assessment is the first stage of this model, which is followed by planning, implementation and evaluation. Other nursing models used in primary health care nursing include the activities of daily living framework (Roper *et al.* 1980) and Orem's model, which emphasises health and views the person as an integrated whole with a motivation to achieve self-care (Orem 1985).

Nursing assessments in primary care have been defined in the past by the dominant demands of the role. For example, district nurses have mostly concentrated on physical dimensions of need, and health visitors on the developmental stages of the child. There is, however, more and more emphasis today in the nursing literature on the importance of holistic and comprehensive assessments, which embrace the following categories of need: orientation, mood, activities of daily living, mobility, occupation, social integration, and economic and environmental factors.

The knowledge base required for holistic and patient-centred assessments is complex in terms of the integration of knowledge of biological sciences, epidemiology, communication skills, clin-ical skills and understanding human behaviour. To a large extent our understanding of this area is limited to a few studies (Luker and Kenrick 1992), and for example Walker's (1994) work, which show that a district nurse's assessment of non-malignant pain has shortcomings in that psycho-social elements are often overlooked. The extent to which issues of mental health and social integration are included in assessments is patchy. This reflects the fact that most practitioners are better at defining and identifying physical health problems; therefore the identification of mental health problems, and particularly depression, often goes undeclared and unrecognised in primary health care (Illife *et al.* 1991, Blanchard *et al.* 1994). It is not surprising if questions which explore older clients' emotional needs have been overlooked in district nursing (Ross and Bower 1995). This raises mental health training issues, particularly in view of the fact that Thomas and Corney (1993) found that 89 per cent of practice nurses in their sample had caseloads which included people with psychological problems.

Assessment and care management in community care

The introduction of assessment and care management into community care is driven by value-for-money considerations, the need to provide integrated and seamless care, and the intent to reflect user and carer concerns in the assessment and delivery of care (see Chapter 1). There are many conceptual and operational difficulties about assessment and care management that exist not only for individual professional groups but also between disciplines and participating agencies. Some of these difficulties include confusion over the definition of case/care management, the role in relation to assessment, referral, decision making, resource allocation, interprofessional and interagency work, confidentiality, and the interpretation of the role in relation to various client groups and settings in community and primary care.

Care management

The term care management originated from case management. During consultation on the policy guidance for community care, case was regarded as demeaning to the individual, and misleading in that it is the care and not the person that is being managed. Both terms are referred to in the literature on this subject, but care management is the preferred term in this book.

The experience of care/case management in the UK is limited. The concept originated in the United States. The only extensively evaluated scheme in Britain is the Kent Community Care Scheme (Challis and Davies 1986), which has been replicated in Gateshead and Darlington. Care management as a concept is subject to widely differing interpretations. Bergen (1992) highlights common themes arising from the literature about care management, such as: normalisation, choice and dignity for individuals; accessibility and advocacy on the part of professionals; and flexibility and innovation on the part of service management.

The principles of care management include:

1. an approach to assessment and the delivery of services based on clients' needs rather than service availability
2. a framework of locally determined objectives and priorities
3. partnership among other agencies
4. partnership with the client and carer
5. information, monitoring, quality assurance and review

The DoH (1991) has described seven core tasks which make up the whole process:

1. publishing information
2. determining levels of assessment
3. assessing need
4. care planning
5. implementing the care plan
6. monitoring services
7. reviewing

The care management process is described in Figure 3.1.

The care manager has been defined as any practitioner who undertakes all or most of the 'core tasks' of care management,

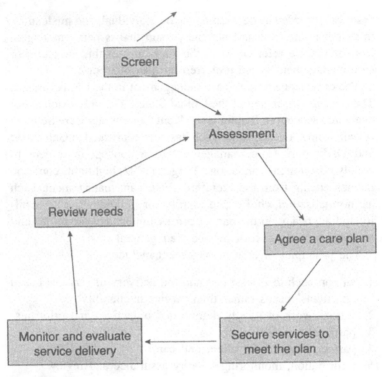

Figure 3.1 Care management process
Source: NHSTD 1994

who may carry budgetary responsibility, but is not involved in any direct service provision. It is intended that the care manager should act as a broker for services across the statutory and independent sectors. It is not expected that the care manager should be involved in direct service delivery, or carry management responsibility. This therefore separates the process of procuring services from delivery, and it is hoped will remove any possibility of conflict of interest. At the present time there are many interpretations of the above, and it is not surprising if there is some confusion over the nature of the role, and how it relates to the notion of the assessor, key worker and co-ordinator.

Assessment in care management is the process of objectively defining needs by the Local Authority. Lewis *et al.* (1995) point out that this encapsulates the tension, unacknowledged in the White Paper, between identifying need and allowing choice on the one hand, and rationing on the other. In other words, there are many potential conflicts arising from needs-led assessment within a resource-finite system that has to employ rationing. Therefore processes have been developed to determine eligibility for assistance against stated policy criteria.

Criteria of eligibility for social care assessment have been agreed by the Local Authority, Health Authority and Family Health Services Authority. This is to ensure that the assessment of need and the services that flow from it meet certain criteria. Information from the Community Care database indicates that in some authorities these have been defined in terms of crisis management, such as avoiding imminent breakdown of care arrangements, risk of abuse or neglect, or requiring help and support with personal care. Other authorities have defined the eligibility criteria more broadly to encompass psycho-social needs, e.g. living alone, presence of serious physical or mental illness, disability or degree of stress unacceptable to person, carer or community. Clearly the thinking, planning and implementation of care management are developing fast and criteria will be modified in the light of experience, resource constraints and the response and pattern of service delivery. (Note: The Community Care Support Force database was funded up to 1995. It was based at the Nuffield Institute for Health Services Research. Its purpose was to disseminate examples of innovative practice in community care.)

The aim of assessment in care management is that it should be a participative process involving the applicant, their carers and other relevant agencies. The policy defines need as the requirements of individuals to enable them to achieve, maintain or restore an acceptable level of social independence or quality of life, as defined by the particular agency or authority (DoH 1990b). Thus need is a personal and relative concept, which is

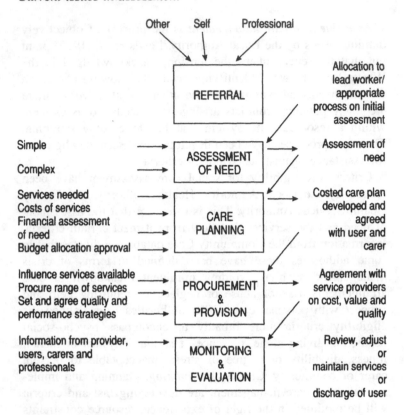

Figure 3.2 Care management – stages and tasks
Source: NHSTD 1993

to be defined and assessed at the local level. Local Authorities have put in place systems to ensure that they can carry out a range of assessments from simple to complex. Some assessments also require specialist skills, for example in mental health or learning disabilities. The way in which assessments are defined and approached has been variously interpreted by different Local Authorities. For example, Wandsworth Borough Council developed the following definitions of the stages and tasks that form their version of an assessment hierarchy:

1. *Simple assessment:* a limited assessment undertaken by either a social worker or an occupational therapist and leading to either:

   - referral for comprehensive assessment, or
   - provision of fixed criteria services such as bus pass, or
   - provision of OT services, or
   - referral to another Local Authority or a voluntary organisation to provide a service, or
   - no service

A simple assessment does not include the completion of the core assessment form.

2. *Core assessment:* an assessment which involves completion of the core assessment form (agreed by the participating agencies) even though in some cases only the appropriate and relevant sections are completed. This information is used to develop the care plan in partnership with the clients and carers wherever possible.

3. *Complex assessment:* a comprehensive assessment which involves other agencies or disciplines in completing additional separate specialist assessments.

4. *Review:* a routine further assessment of an established care package to check it continues to meet assessed needs.

5. *Reassessment:* an additional and urgent core or complex assessment triggered by a significant change in the client's circumstances.

Care management and nursing interface – some practice examples

The White Paper (DoH 1989c) was not prescriptive about who should be the care manager. It suggested that care managers could be drawn from professionals with backgrounds in social services, occupational therapy, nursing and general practice. Thus it offers exciting opportunities for nurses to develop aspects of the role. In a survey of Health Authorities, however, Bergen

(1994) found that the extent to which care management policies had been adopted, and the involvement of primary health care nursing, were both patchy, and mostly identified community psychiatric nursing. Bergen's study was carried out before the growth of initiatives that appeared in the wake of the delayed implementation date for community care in 1993.

The review of innovations carried out in 1994 (Ross and Elliott 1995) identified several interesting examples of mostly district nursing involvement in care management, e.g. developing assessment forms and criteria for assessment in collaboration with social services, and in some instances even in consultation with users and carers.

The care management project reported by Bourke-Dowling (1994) demonstrated that assessment by district nurses for limited social care needs did not involve significant changes for the district nurse but increased role credibility, job satisfaction and understanding of social services' role and reduced unnecessary visits to the client. The database on community care held by the Nuffield Institute for Health has evidence of new organisational models. In some cases district nurses have been seconded to work in social services to carry out full care manager responsibilities, and in Northumberland there has been a pilot of budget holding by a social worker seconded to the primary health care team. Other Local Authorities such as Oxfordshire plan to recruit staff from a variety of backgrounds, including district and psychiatric nursing, to be care managers. There are some difficulties with this model, because of lack of clarification as to whether the district nurse, for example, should work purely as a purchaser (organising and monitoring packages of care) or should provide nursing care as well.

Assessment and the interface between community nursing, general practice and social services – a case study

An evaluation of a joint planning initiative that piloted care management within the context of social services, general practice and community nursing has just been completed by one of the authors (Ross and Tissier 1994) and will be reported on in some detail here. The study was an evaluation of a pilot project set up to build on the pivotal role of primary health care services in community care, particularly in relation to elderly and physically disabled people. The project was designed to focus on the GP practice as the setting for assessment and care management initiatives and to explore the benefits of closely co-ordinating the assessment of need for health and social care at an early stage in the referral of clients with complex needs. A social worker (care manager) was attached to two general practices and worked with a district nurse (care manager) to focus on the process and systems of care management from referral to closure; the integration of health and social care; and the views, concerns and values of practitioners, managers, users and carers.

The method involved collection of referral information held by social services and community nursing, scrutiny of case records, documentary analysis and qualitative interviews with professionals, users and carers.

The findings from this study reveal a number of important and interesting issues that exemplify some of the dilemmas surrounding assessment and care management in community and primary health care, and at the boundary of health and social care. The operational issues, and the difficulties of making care management work, emerged through the interview data and the analysis of referral patterns. The themes of communication and information flow were identified frequently in relation to the user, general practitioner, social worker (care manager) and the district nurse (care manager). The value of the social worker (care manager) as a single point of contact was emphasised by the GPs and the district nurse, because it served to facilitate joint visiting, provided the opportunity for feedback and avoided unnecessary duplication in assessment. Although there were a number of resource constraints that limited the district nurse's care management role in this project, an excellent working relationship between the district nurse and social worker developed, which promoted mutual understanding of other working systems. Because the community nursing and social services information systems were not compatible, however, it was not possible for a case on the social services' database to be allocated in full to the district nurse, even where it had been agreed that she was the most appropriate professional to assume the care manager role. Therefore there was no easy way of sharing information. Furthermore, there was some reluctance on the part of some sections of social services to accept the authority of the district nurse as care manager. Finally, the study confirmed that the needs of older people and the disabled are frequently varied and seldom fall neatly within the remit of any one of the caring agencies. The importance of sharing assessment information and co-ordinating care is critical to avoid duplication.

Summary of issues

As Lewis *et al.* (1995) point out, most of the implementation and reviews of assessment in care management have to date been driven by concerns for the elderly. Other client groups such as children do not fit so easily into these models. This may explain why the practice examples described above come from district nursing rather than health visiting. In spite of all the work done by planners, managers and practitioners across all agencies, there are still many difficult questions that remain unanswered. There is the difficulty of involving general practitioners successfully in care management (Leedham and Wistow 1992), and issues of accountability, resources, shared records and confidentiality. Finally, it is important that systems are developed that seek to clarify and do not merely add more layers of bureaucracy, to the disadvantage of users and carers.

Community care policies present nurses in primary care with opportunities to feed their knowledge and experience of health-needs assessment into the care management and assessment process. There are organisational and professional barriers to doing this. Innovations in policy and practice and local solutions to the problems need to be shared.

Assessment and the GP health check

The 1990 GP Contract made it a requirement that GPs carry out an annual assessment of their registered patient population over 75 years. The focus of the assessment is on social needs, mobility, mental health, sensory needs, continence, functional performance and medication.

This health assessment initiative of people over 75 years old, or screening as it is sometimes incorrectly known, is based on the assumption that there are unmet needs among the elderly in the community. This idea largely originated from important work done in the 1960s, which showed that in screened elderly populations a high prevalence of unreported physical, social and psychological problems existed (Williamson *et al.* 1964, Townsend and Wedderburn 1965). More recently, the evidence that the elderly are underconsulters has been challenged. Ebrahim *et al.* (1984) point out that non-consulting elderly people are on the whole a fit and low-risk group. In view of the fact that there is little contemporary evidence for the effectiveness of screening elderly people in terms of health and economic benefits (Freer 1985, Freer 1987), a blanket screening policy of elderly people is probably inappropriate. There is some consensus that it should be replaced with a system of opportunistic case finding, combined with targeted assessment of people in at-risk groups (Illife *et al.* 1991).

In spite of the reservations based on research findings, the current contractual expectations are for a universal and annual health check. In a national survey carried out by Chew, Wilkin and Glendinning (1994), it was found that a variety of methods were in use in general practice, varying from opportunistic doctor-led assessment during a consultation to practice nurse-led recall and assessment and, less frequently, assessments carried out by practice-attached health visitors or district nurses. Further, it was found that a variety of different checklists or interview schedules had been adopted.

It is important that the assessment documentation system selected should be user friendly and comprehensive across the main domains of assessment, and should ideally fit into existing record systems such as the Lloyd George envelope. The main problem with the checklist format is that it does not offer a standardised way of asking questions. Therefore the information may be different depending on who the interviewer is, and the way in which the questions are asked. In order to elicit the patients' concerns the interviewer requires good communication skills, knowledge and expertise in the care of the elderly and a positive view of ageing.

The Royal College of General Practitioners has recommended a three-stage assessment framework (Williams and Wallace 1993). The first stage aims to identify health and social problems at an early stage. The second stage assessment is undertaken if a problem has been identified using the routine practice-based methods of problem solving. The recommendation for the third stage is to use the Royal College of Physicians' suite of assessment instruments (SAFE). It seems, however, that the implications of these recommendations have not been fully thought through, particularly in terms of the feasibility of linking these assessment strategies with the core assessment in care management, which perhaps explains the disappointingly low uptake nationally of this system (Chew *et al.* 1994).

Who should do the health check?

Part of the debate about the costs of the health check of older people concerns who should do it. This begs the question of who in the primary care team sees this sort of work as valuable and important. There is an ambivalence among members of the primary care team about who should be responsible for the assessment of older people. In one study the majority of primary care team members thought the health visitor was the most appropriate health professional, although half the health visitors themselves disagreed, seeing their priorities as being with the 0–5 year olds (Tremellen and Jones 1989). Most studies have in fact identified the practice nurse as doing the majority of the assessments (Brown *et al.* 1992, Tremellen 1992), with doctors doing some, rare inputs from health visitors and district nurses and, in some cases, assessments being carried out by volunteers (Carpenter and Demopoulos 1990).

Given that practice nurses are key players in this work and that compared to general practitioners they are more positive about the value of health assessments (Chew *et al.* 1994), it is of some concern that they often lack suitable training in care of the elderly (Brown *et al.* 1992, Ross *et al.* 1994). Brown *et al.* (1992) found that one-third of practice nurses in their study had had no training at all. This is supported by Chew *et al.*'s (1994) finding that when they had guidelines relating to assessment, these were often limited in scope, and focused on recall methods rather than clinical guidelines.

The training issues are related to the philosophy and approach to assessment. Perkins (1991) describes the spirit that should be behind elderly assessment as being about eliciting the patients' concerns rather than imposing a professionally defined view of need. She advocates using a version of a biographical approach as a way of solving problems. Clearly this requires assessors to have not only a positive view of ageing and a knowledge base of elderly care, but also sophisticated and sensitive interviewing and communication skills. For example, poorly conceived questions may undermine someone's coping strategies or raise unrealistic expectations about what can be offered. It is important that nurses are aware of the dilemmas that follow when a need for a service is identified and the service is known to be rationed. As well as raising expectations for services that are in practice non-existent, there is the danger of raising unrealistic expectations about health and recovery. On the other hand, an inappropriate offer of help may undermine, for some people, the integrity of their independence.

Ethical issues

The universal health check raises a number of important ethical issues that should remain at the centre of the debate. The first point is that patients have a right to be assessed by skilled and motivated professionals. There is no doubt that practice nurses need and want better training. The politics of practice nurse training are complex and confused, however, and lie between the GP as employer, central government and nursing professional bodies. Secondly, elderly people have a right to choose whether or not they are assessed. Thirdly, they have a right to the information collected, particularly when assessment of need may not lead to the offer of a service. Finally, it should be no surprise to anyone reading this chapter that one of the consequences of this new focus on assessment is that there is a danger of overassessment and duplication between agencies.

Summary of issues

The health assessment of older people in general practice raises several issues. In the first place there is the question of whether or not targeting health checks would be more desirable and cost effective. Secondly, it would seem that the skills of the nursing team are not being used most appropriately, in that the nurses who are trained in elderly care (district nurses and health visitors) are on the whole not doing the work. Even if they do not have the time to take it on, surely this is an opportunity for informal peer group teaching or mentoring to take place within practices to promote skill sharing. Finally, there is still work to be done on thinking through how the results of the health check could feed into the parallel developments of community care assessments by the use of a standardised assessment. This is discussed in the next section.

Standardised assessment

The focus on assessment has involved considerable professional energy in developing assessment instruments to suit the particular needs of nursing, general practice and social work, as well as secondary care. Inevitably there is the danger of reinventing the wheel, and endless duplication of effort developing assessment instruments that are not validated or connected with other systems. Finally, both care management and the over-75-year-old health check are generating a huge amount of data that is limited in usefulness, because of lack of standardisation of methods.

In early 1992 the Royal College of Physicians and the British Geriatric Society led a multi-disciplinary workshop that set out to reach a consensus on a 'basket of measures' for the assessment of the major domains of need in the elderly – activities of daily living, orientation, mood, quality of life and social need. This is known as Standardised Assessment Scales for Elderly People (SAFE). The workshop agreed on a number of benefits of standardised scales – described as the 10 Cs (Dickinson and Mayer 1995) and detailed in Box 3.2.

Box 3.2 The potential uses of data from standardised assessments (the 10 Cs)

Clinical care:	to encourage best practice in screening, assessment, ongoing management and discharge planning
Clinical records:	to assist in the sharing of assessments and setting of joint care goals
Communication:	to provide a common language of care to aid communication between professionals, patients, families, carers and the different sectors of care
Coding:	to allow coding, capture and computerisation of assessment data

Comparison:	to permit routine outcome assessment, and, as a casemix measure, assist in the interpretation of outcome comparisons
Collaboration:	to facilitate collaboration between disciplines and the sharing of workloads by eliminating duplication in assessment
Cost-effectiveness:	to facilitate the routine evaluation of new services and the execution of systematic overviews of clinical trials
Contracting:	to form a basis for defining the clientele and activities of health services for elderly people
Community health:	to help in the aggregation of data on the health status of elderly people from diverse sources
Clinical audit:	to streamline the clinical audit of the care of elderly people

Source: Dickinson 1994

As a result of the workshops a suite of assessment instruments were recommended and published in a report by the SAFE working group (Royal College of Physicians/British Geriatric Society 1992) and further discussed by Philp (1994). They included the Barthel Activity of Daily Living Index, the Abbreviated Mental Test, the Geriatric Depression Scale and the Philadelphia Morale Scale. Although these scales have been used and tested for reliability and feasibility in research studies, there are few examples of their usefulness in routine clinical use. It was the question of their feasibility, interpretation and usefulness that the SAFE study group set out to assess in eight different clinical settings of elderly care. The author carried out one of these studies with district nurses in primary care (Ross and Bower 1995). The following section briefly describes this study, the application of standard measures of assessment in district nursing and the benefits for joint working.

The rationale for this study was to assess the extent to which instruments agreed by an interprofessional working group were transferable to, and feasible for use by, district nurses with elderly people at home. Forty people aged 65 years or over, recently discharged from hospital and in the care of district nurses, were interviewed at home using the recommended scales and in addition an adapted social check list. Feasibility was assessed in terms of the time taken, acceptability to patient and carer, and the extent to which the outcome of the research assessment was in agreement with the district nurse's judgement.

The mean time taken to complete the scales was 39.3 minutes, which was more than twice as long as reported in the hospital based studies. This may be because elderly people are more inclined to answer questions discursively in their own homes compared to the public arena of the hospital bed with only a curtain for privacy. Given the comprehensive nature of information collected, however, this is not an unreasonable use of time in district nursing practice. The majority of patients valued the time spent on the interviews, and none of the carers expressed reservations. There was a high scoring on the depression scale, and questions aimed at eliciting extent of depression and quality of life were the most difficult to ask, and were often not completed. Given that depression among elderly people often goes unrecognised, however, it is important that nurses have acceptable measures for its assessment. This is an area that many of the patients were grateful for the time to explore, and an area that is often overlooked in professional assessment.

This study demonstrates that adopting standard measures of assessment in district nursing is feasible and useful, in that domains of need previously ignored are included. Moreover, the wider implications of this type of common approach to assessment have advantages in that the assessment data can translate and be acceptable to other disciplines and be used across the interface of primary and secondary care. Ultimately, common information systems could be developed based on a common and agreed language of assessment. This would greatly facilitate the seamless care that current policy has defined as desirable.

Conclusion

Clearly there are many difficult issues around assessment highlighted by this discussion of the needs of older people. The GP health check is generating a huge amount of data on the over-75-year-old population, but it is of limited use because there have been no common, standardised systematic methods used in collecting the information. It is vital that standardised systems are set up in general practice to connect with care management and the demands to define population needs, so that services can be offered appropriately for older people.

Chapter 4
Interprofessional work

Summary

This chapter aims to discuss the link between developing policies for interprofessional work in primary health care and the extent to which these ideas are reflected in practice. The chapter seeks to clarify the overlapping terms of interprofessional, teamwork and collaboration, and to discuss the empirical research carried out in the field of primary health care. The concept of working together in primary health care gives rise to some important tensions for planners, managers and practitioners, such as multi-skilling, the health and social care divide, the inherent conflict between collaboration and the internal market, user choice, fragmentation and integration. Some of the important arenas for interprofessional work involving nurses in primary care are selected for detailed discussion.

Introduction

The importance of teamwork for the effective delivery of primary health care has been a recurring theme in policy statements over the last 15 years. There is a generally held belief that working together, like apple pie, is a good thing. Despite the rhetoric about teamwork in primary care over the last twenty years there has been little in the way of evidence to substantiate the view that collaboration leads to either health gains or improved patient outcomes. Therefore it is timely to reframe the questions now. What is the exact meaning of teamwork? What are the constraints to achieving it? And what understanding do we have of its benefits? This chapter draws from the literature on teamwork in primary health care, and integrates it with issues arising from nursing in order to refine future questions for practice and research.

Historical and policy background

It is not the purpose here to trace the detail of this strand of policy, rather to outline the context for a discussion of the meaning, interpretation and application of interprofessional work for nurses in primary health care. Primary health care and teamwork have been promoted in successive policy documents, with a particular emphasis on health promotion. This began in the mid-1970s, with the recognition by the then Labour government of the need for a shift from institutional and acute care to meet the challenges of a growing elderly population and life-style related diseases in the community. The intention was that this reorientation of care should be led by primary health care teams, in which nurses had a key role (DHSS 1976, DHSS 1977). The Harding report (DHSS 1981b) favoured strengthening the primary care team to deal with these challenges, and it made some important recommendations on multi-disciplinary education for trainee nurses and doctors, which have largely remained on the shelf.

The Conservative administration of the last 15 years has not only reinforced the policies for community care (DHSS 1981b), inner-city primary care (London Health Consortium 1981) and health promotion (DHSS 1987), but it also introduced a new way of looking at service efficiency and effectiveness in the context of an internal market (DoH 1989b). The last ten years in particular have seen a shift in policy from the welfare state and the public monopoly of welfare towards the development of internal markets in health care (discussed in more detail in Chapter 1). Arguably the introduction of GP fundholding has marked a new departure for interprofessional relations. The introduction of GP fundholders with their new freedoms to employ health and welfare staff, and from 1993 the right to contract community nursing services from local Community Units and Trusts, has meant that the fundholding practice team has the potential to become a powerful providing and purchasing unit. This reflects explicit government policy that states that the GP and the primary care team should become the pivot of health care and drive the shift in the balance of care from the secondary sector (NHSME 1993a).

Definitions and the theoretical framework for interprofessional work

There are many questions raised by this emphasis on teamwork in primary care. The first is, how far has our understanding of teamwork progressed over the last 20 years? It is perhaps a reflection of the complex conceptual, structural and professional issues that lie at its roots that have resulted in slow progress of understanding, interpretation and implementation in practice.

There is considerable conceptual confusion over the meaning and relationship between collaboration at an interagency, inter-professional and interpersonal level, not least because of the complicated interweaving of theoretical ideas and academic traditions that influence and drive the various key contributors and enthusiasts in this field, for example social policy (Leathard 1994); sociology of professionals in relation to health policy (Owens and Carrier 1995); organisational psychology (Poulton and West 1994); and interpersonal and group relations (Meek and Pietroni 1993). The focus of this chapter is drawn from a mixture of social policy, to explain the pressures for inter-professional work, and the sociology of professions to address the opportunities, constraints, processes and relationships that pertain in the field of primary health care nursing.

Leathard (1994) describes the terminological quagmire of alter-native terms that are used variously to describe working and learning together. She has developed a taxonomy that differentiates between terms that are *concept based* such as interdisciplinary, multi-disciplinary; terms that are *process based* such as teamwork, collaboration, co-ordination and integration; and finally *agency-based* terms such as interagency, intersectoral and alliance. Often there is interchangeable use of terms such as multi-disciplinary and interprofessional. In this chapter the preferred terms are interprofessional and collaboration. The prefix 'inter' rather than 'multi' is preferred, because the former denotes interactive working whereas the latter merely differentiates quantitatively from a single discipline. The term interprofessional, however, as indeed all the alternatives, exposes a fundamental and unresolved problem, in that by definition it excludes patients, carers and health workers who do not hold a professional qualification.

Teamwork has been defined as: 'a group of persons who are trained in the use of different tools and concepts, among whom there is an organised division of labour' (Luski 1958: 10). The basics of team work, in the early seminal work by Margaret Gilmore and her colleagues (Gilmore *et al.* 1974), were seen to be a common purpose, distinctive role and expertise, with some defining leadership. The term collaboration seems to be gaining popularity over team work, perhaps because it allows for different levels of working together, and does not exclude participation by the user. The notion of team work presupposes some form of democratic organisation of health care professionals, which nevertheless depends on collaboration for effectiveness. Gregson *et al.* (1991) suggest that by focusing on collaboration it is possible to explore perceptions, values, expectations, assumptions and behaviours as well as structures. Collaboration is therefore a more useful concept in the analysis of the policies and practice of primary health care.

The theoretical context for interprofessional work examined here includes ideas from the sociology of the professions and notions of professional dominance and social control. Professional dominance describes the effect that the medical profession has had on restricting the practices and subordinating the work of other health professionals (Friedson 1970, Etzioni 1969). This notion has been applied to district nurses by Hockey (1979), Bowling (1981) and Ross (1988). The dominance of health workers by the medical profession is arguably part of the wider medicalisation of society. The second concept, social control (Zola 1975), is understood to be a consequence of the differential relationship between patient and doctor in terms of status, power and knowledge. It may be expressed as the patient's lack of information and perceived helplessness, contrasted with the doctor's expertise. Clearly both these notions of professional dominance and social control function in a hierarchical system of health care. Working collaboratively, however, presupposes a flat structure with shared objectives and access to shared information (Ross 1988). The question that will be returned to in the examination of the following key issues is whether or not this is a realistic and feasible expectation, given the structural constraints to achieving collaboration in primary health care.

Much of the analysis of team work has ignored the user's role apart from teams offering open access to the user (Anderson 1969, Ross 1980). It is interesting that despite the lip service paid to users in current policy statements, they have not been moved centre stage. Sixteen years ago, Webb and Hobdell (1980) argued that the failure of teamwork was due to a failure to recognise two legitimating principles of 'consumer sovereignty' and the 'authority of relevance'. The first describes the patient as an active rather than a passive recipient of care. The second principle, the 'authority of relevance', refers to the importance of valuing information equally from different team members, whatever their position in the hierarchy. Muriel Skeet illustrated these ideas graphically by what she called the pie concept:'each member of the team is a wedge of a different size according to the problem of the patient . . . always the patient and his family have a wedge' (Skeet 1978: 29).

More recently Biggs (1993) challenges interprofessional work for its tendency to exclude the user. He argues that it is vital to look at this interface between the user and the provider in order to refocus attention on new pathways and methods of care provision.

Is collaboration a reality in primary health care?

This question has been asked many times over the last 20 years. More specifically the questions raised are: to what extent does team work improve co-ordination, enhance the quality of care, indeed who benefits? Most studies have focused on the process and the nature of the collaboration between health professionals rather than patient outcomes. Undoubtedly this is important and embraces the shared values, shared goals and 'also the shared meanings about priorities, good practice and quality assurance' (Owens and Carrier 1995). For example, the early work of Gilmore, Bruce and Hunt (1974) provided descriptive information on communication patterns between general practitioners, health visitors and district nurses. Communication was seen to be haphazard, unsystematic and fleeting. The majority of teams had no method of written communication and most had no meetings. Inadequate opportunities for formal meetings have been confirmed by Woods *et al.* (1983) and McClure (1984). Gregson *et al.* (1991) looked at the collaboration of doctor–nurse pairs and identified that a shared base and stable working relationships were important factors in promoting collaboration. This study was important because it developed a methodology for measuring indices of working together, and it also served as the base for further descriptive research of the discrepancies in understanding and perception among members of primary health care teams in 20 practices in Northumberland (Hutchinson and Gordon 1992).

That there is a 'feel good' factor for professionals working together is undoubted. But is this in itself sufficient justification for team organisation? Recently some authors have argued that 'we need to move on from process to look at ways of intervening to deliver specific outcomes' (Pearson and Jones 1994). Jones (1992) suggests that the concept of the team will be better understood in the context of the task it is performing. It is likely that the task arises from the relationship between professionals, but focusing on the task will permit better understanding of the relationship, and more importantly define the outcome. For example, professionals providing terminal care at home, or the practice team devising a new protocol with an audit tool for the management of asthmatic children, will be able to define the objectives, the individual roles and contribution, and the agreed measure of outcome. There are some examples of this happening in primary health care. For example, an occupational therapist working in a multi-disciplinary team in West Lothian initiated a motor neurone support group, which aimed to enhance co-ordination, minimise duplication on assessment and increase the understanding of roles (Anderson 1993).

The murky world of interprofessional work in primary health care

Although a focus on tasks is a helpful way of reframing the difficulties of interprofessional work it will not remove the fundamental and structural barriers to team work in primary care identified by Dingwall (1980). These, he argued, arose from the different employment characteristics of general practitioners – as the independent contractors – in contrast to the Health Authority-employed health visitors and district nurses, and the practice-employed practice nurses. In addition to this are the constraints of professional status, education level and gender. As well as the interface between primary health care nurses and general practitioners, there is the relationship with social services and the Local Authority. There has been considerable recent discussion of the different organisational structures, priorities, philosophies and funding mechanisms that exist between Health and Local Authorities.

The following are examples from practice of what Schon would call the low swamplands of professional uncertainty (Schon 1992) – in other words, where there is role confusion over specific tasks in primary care. It is because the patterns of these tasks are so unstable, and the solutions often organisational, that they evoke strong feelings and frustration among the professionals and often the patients involved. In these cases professionals have the opportunity, through working together, to reshape roles by reorganisation and rationalisation.

Practice examples of interprofessional disputes

Immunisation of children   This is carried out either in child health clinics or the GP's surgery. In the latter there is often disagreement over who should do it: general practitioner, health visitor, practice nurse or district nurse? The question is not about competence, but resources. The roots of the conflict go back to who feels they own the patient and who benefits. Immunisations are reimbursed on an item of service fee payable to the practice. Health visitors are concerned to monitor the immunisation take-up of children on their caseloads, and perceive themselves as professionally accountable for this area of work. Additional questions arise about who should do immunisations in the home. If the drive is to increase immunisation rates to meet the practice target, is this a job for the health visitor or the practice nurse?

Social baths   In the past district nurses provided this service. Now, because of financial stringency and the requirement on Health Authorities to be accountable only for spending on health needs, this role has shifted to social services. Do social services staff miss opportunities for health promotion and the early detection of problems? Are they adequately trained? Do users like it?

Over-75-year-old health checks   The requirement to carry out an annual health check of all patients over 75 years was introduced in the 1990 GP Contract. This is intended to be a medical and social assessment. Given that the income is directed at general practice, district nurses are ambivalent about doing this work, and it is not cost effective for GPs to do it routinely. The following questions arise. Which nurse in primary health care has the knowledge base, time and motivation? Is it suitable work for a trained lay worker? Do patients like it, and is it cost effective?

The provision of nursing equipment and aids to daily living to patients in their own homes   In theory the funding and provision of the former come from the Health Authority and of the latter from the Local Authority. In practice there are problems due to poor communication between district nurses and social services and to different priorities of need and caring. The patient experiences a system that is patchy, inequitable and unresponsive, and one where relevant and helpful information is sparse (Ross and Campbell 1992). There are many questions arising. Who should assess for incontinence aids when the problem is a long-term one? If a commode is needed urgently, should a district nurse collect it herself? Whose responsibility is it that aids and equipment are unused in patients' homes? Who should assess for a commode – a district nurse or an occupational therapist? Should patients know the availability of aids/equipment? Who is responsible?

Current issues and debates in interprofessional care

Interprofessional work raises many interesting issues, some of which are selected for more detailed discussion below.

Interprofessionalism as a precursor to deprofessionalising health care

Carrier and Kendall (1995) identify a tension between, on the one hand, conceptualising multi-professional work as a co-operative enterprise in which traditional forms and divisions of professional knowledge and authority are retained, and on the other hand taking the more radical view of interprofessional work, which 'implies a willingness to share and indeed give up exclusive claims to specialised knowledge and authority, if the needs of clients can be met more efficiently by other professional groups' (Carrier and Kendall 1995: 10). This crystallises the opportunities and the risks of promoting interprofessional work. The opportunity is there for all professionals to understand better their core of knowledge and expertise and the extent to which it is discrete from and overlapping with that of others in the team. For example, a district nurse has in her repertoire the skills to help patients and carers to understand and cope with the consequences of chronic disease such as multiple sclerosis. The GP assesses the need for referral, management of medication, and secondary problems. They both continuously share their observations of the patient, exchange information about changes in individual management, and on an ongoing basis adapt the care plan accordingly.

The risks are that the areas of role overlap are seen by some as redundant, with a 'minimum critical specification' (Usherwood 1993). This argument can be extrapolated to a view that in the interests of maximum efficiency anyone can substitute for anyone else, therefore paving the way for a multi-skilled worker to replace professional expertise. Again taking the example of chronic disease, it could be argued that a significant proportion of the role of the occupational therapist, physiotherapist and district nurse be carried out by a suitably trained and multi-skilled health professional. Therefore, paradoxically, arguments for precise definitions of professional boundaries to clarify working relationships may unwittingly be used to dismantle the uniqueness of professional roles and weaken the authority of professions in a process of deprofessionalisation towards the lowest common denominator of multi-skilling. It is not surprising then that for some the blurring of boundaries means loss of boundaries, and makes room for a kind of professional paranoia, or as Schon (1992) suggests, a crisis in professional confidence. This must be guarded against by constantly reviewing professional roles at the interface with the patient.

Continuity of care and a seamless service

An overarching aim of the NHS and community care reforms is the policy intention to work towards seamless and co-ordinated care. Clearly in a system of care delivery with a diversity of providers, ranging from health and social care to the independent and voluntary sectors, it is vital to pay attention to mechanisms of joint working. The implementation of the Community Care

Act in 1993 emphasised the key strategies of care management, assessment and joint working between social and health care agencies in order to deliver co-ordinated and seamless care. More specifically the Local Authority lead role in community care has required collaboration with Community Health Units/Trusts to clarify the role and responsibility of community nurses in priority setting, needs assessment, care planning and resource allocation. Since central government was careful not to be prescriptive about how the policy should be implemented at local level, it is not surprising that there has been some considerable activity and diversity in developing collaborative projects around care management and assessment. The emphasis in this section is on the issues relating to interprofessional work, while care management and assessment are discussed in Chapter 3.

The impetus for the interprofessional work coming from the community care reforms has been in terms of developing jointly agreed criteria for the assessment of health and social need. This has resulted, in some areas, in the development of a core assessment tool, and shared care plans held by the user. Examples of this sort of initiative include a pilot project in South Bedfordshire (Pick 1992); the involvement of district nurses in assessment and care management working with social services and based in a general practice (Ross and Tissier 1994); the development of a district nurse care management role with the elderly physically disabled in Hertfordshire (Bourke-Dowling 1994); secondment of community nurses to social services in Hampshire and the development of agreed definitions and shared assessment protocols (Korczak 1993).

These exciting projects demonstrate positive evidence of working together between professionals and across agencies. There are, however, many lessons that are emerging from the experience of these initiatives. On the positive side, innovative models of interagency and interprofessional work have been documented, with district nurses being involved in new approaches to needs-led assessment, better understanding the role and function of other agencies, pooling knowledge of local resources and enabling people to remain in their own homes. There are, however, major structural difficulties that stand in the way of true implementation of the policy. The root of the problem lies in the separation of funding of health and social care. This means that the potential for a district nurse to play a full role in care management is diminished by the organisational and funding barriers. In other words, a district nurse care manager is practising within the policy remit of one organisation (Local Authority) while being accountable to another (Health Authority). In practice this means that some professionals within social services have been unwilling to accept the authority of the district nurse assessment, therefore restricting the scope of the nursing assessment. There have been difficulties encountered in breaking down barriers between different work cultures, with consequences in changing roles, which have sometimes resulted in fears of role erosion among social workers, home care organisers, occupational therapists and district nurses. The important issue around accountability for assessment, and ultimately resourcing, has been responded to by new contractual models such as secondment and joint and full appointment of district nursing staff to social services teams. Many of the initiatives have identified the need for additional training on the policies, roles and functions of the different organisations, so that social services and nursing staff can fulfil the requirements of the community care legislation.

Conflict between interprofessional work and the competitive thrust of the internal market

Current policy suggests an inherent paradox between on the one hand exhortation for increased interagency and interprofessional working in order to increase effectiveness and responsiveness of the service, and on the other hand pressure to bid successfully for service contracts. This means that the system is subjected to conflicting tensions of push and pull. The main point here is that conflicts arise when the motivation to work interprofessionally is geared more towards securing business and contracts than in the interests of the patient. In primary health care a consultant obstetrician working in antenatal care in a GP surgery may have a tendency to be motivated by the need to maintain his contract with the GP. Outreach nursing teams for stroke rehabilitation will endeavour to work with the core primary health care team, but inevitably motivation in an internal market is to secure business and ultimately perhaps draw funding away from generic workers such as district nurses.

A cult of interprofessionalism or consumer choice?

> *Professionals are a conspiracy against the laity.*
> (*The Doctor's Dilemma*, Bernard Shaw 1911 – Act 1)

There is a real danger of replacing one form of professional dominance, described earlier, with the team becoming a form of interprofessional club. This is overstating the case, but the point to be made here is that the user tends to be on the edge of the team rather than being centre stage as advocated by Webb and Hobdell (1980). In an earlier study of aids and equipment in the community it was found that the patients and carers were intensely frustrated by a lack of information that reflected the gulf between two parts of a dysfunctioning system (Ross and Campbell 1992). This resonates with Leathard's (1994) question: 'how far does interprofessional collaboration increase patient choice?' The study of community nursing innovations (Ross and Elliott 1995) showed that consumer-focused services have mostly developed in response to the need for increased information. Given that poor and absent information is a common criticism by users, there is perhaps an opportunity for the primary health care team to undertake further work to which all can undoubtedly contribute.

Effectiveness and evaluation of interprofessional practice

Interprofessional work was criticised earlier as not being outcome focused. An opportunity to redress this is presented by the recent work on developing clinical guidelines. This work has developed from audit initiatives in primary care that were initially uni-disciplinary and in the main funded for general practice through the Medical Audit Advisory Groups (MAGS) with the exception of some central government audit money, which was allocated through regions and was made available for competing bids from nurses and Professions Allied to Medicine (PAMs). The focus of this has changed to multi-disciplinary audit and multi-disciplinary guidelines. This gives nurses in primary care the opportunity to contribute to the development of guidelines for practice, and also to contribute to the evaluation of the effectiveness of these through the multi-disciplinary audit programme. This is in its early stages, but paves the way to truly affect practice and patient care by tailoring the work of the team to the needs of the user. It also offers the potential to involve the user in developing the guidelines, for example the management of people with dementia, leg ulcers and osteoarthritis.

Is teamwork a threat to personal care?

A question that often creeps into the discussion of interprofessional care is, how far does the team approach threaten the individual professional's personal and continuing relationship with the patient? A related question is, if a patient confides in one team member should this information become the public property of the team? There are no bland answers to these questions. There are undoubtedly times when the individual relationship is in itself therapeutic – this is something that all professionals experience at some time with patients, and is of equally central importance for the district nurse and occupational therapist as for the doctor. It would seem that the point here is that there is a continuum of personal care and collaboration for any patient, and that this varies in unique and subtle ways for individual patients and individual professionals and teams, depending on the needs.

Evaluation of collaboration

There are huge problems in measuring the effectiveness of a team approach even when intervention is limited to a single condition, because of the difficulties of controlling for confounding variables. Measuring the outcomes of collaboration is at the present time imprecise, and intervention studies in this field in the UK are limited.

Arenas of interprofessional work in primary health care

Many arenas of interprofessional work have already been discussed, such as joint assessment, care management and the development of multi-disciplinary clinical guidelines. Other important ones include healthy alliances, health promotion, hospital discharges, the changing frame of the primary health care team and, at an interagency level, joint commissioning. There are other important areas such as child protection, mental health care, and client-based issues such as palliative care, elder abuse, for which it is possible to identify principles rather than details of care in this chapter.

Healthy alliances and health promotion

The first ever government health policy demonstrated a policy shift from disease management and an illness service to an emphasis on health and its promotion. The *Health of the Nation* document identifies targets for health and is outcome based (see Chapter 1). To be effective it requires an interprofessional approach and work across agencies, sometimes known as healthy alliances.

Beattie (1994) points out that it is striking that each major professional group claims that health promotion lies at the foundation of their work, and it is an important element in the rethinking of professional roles. This supports Bunton and Macdonald's (1992) view that the new public health movement requires a realignment of professional loyalties and ultimately a reframing of professional identities. Health visiting is an example of this, illustrated by the debate on the reorientation of their role from child health to public health. The role of practice nurses has been recently re-defined by the health promotion requirement of the GP Contract, and district nurses need to consider their health promotion focus through the process of needs analysis and target groups. The process of needs analysis, as explained in Chapter 2, is currently unsophisticated, but will be made a requirement by commissioning agencies.

This section focuses on some of the successes of interprofessional work in health promotion. The most notable experiment has been the Local Organising Team Workshops (LOTS) scheme of health promotion organised by the Health Education Authority. This is a residential three-day scheme for GPs and their teams to work together and agree an action plan to prevent coronary heart disease. A secondary objective of these workshops is to increase interprofessional understanding (Jones 1990). Spratley's (1989) evaluation shows that in 159 out of 161 practices taking part, both health promotion activities and enhanced teamwork were still in evidence two years later.

Other successes identified in the study of community nursing innovations are school nurses working with teachers, parents and school children to promote positive health messages (Atmarow *et al.* 1993); health promotion taken to the clients in a leisure centre that required working with community health professionals and the commercial sector (Thomas 1993a); cardiac rehabilitation and continuity of care for patients on discharge, which has reduced the number of inpatient days to five for an uncomplicated myocardial infarction (Evans 1994); and a sexual health and contraception clinic (Streetwise) specifically for the under-16 age group in an inner city. The latter uses a multi-agency approach that allows staff to refer between youth workers, counsellors and medical practitioners (Packham 1993).

As well as the above community-based health promotion initiatives, practice nurses are in a key role to carry out the health promotion requirements of the GP Contract. The sudden increase in numbers of practice nurses in the early 1990s reflected the fact that practice nurses were taken on to carry out new patient health checks, over-75-year-old health checks and chronic disease management (for further discussion see Chapter 7).

Hospital discharge

Many research studies carried out over the last 20 years have revealed problems experienced by patients during and after discharge from hospital (Victor and Vetter 1988, Williams and Fitton 1991), and that community services are often given short notice and inadequate information of discharge (Savill and Bartholomew 1994). Cost effectiveness of the system, reflected in the pressure on throughput and early discharge, and the requirements of the Community Care Act to ensure consultation with relevant members of the caring team from health and social services, mean that this is an increasingly important arena for interprofessional decision making. Recommendations from a recent research study are for a named member of the multi-disciplinary team to be responsible for co-ordinating discharge arrangements, including information relevant to the discharge, assessments done and services contacted (Tierney *et al.* 1994).

The primary health care team

Throughout this chapter there have been references to the primary health care team. The early work on team work came largely from primary health care, and today it is a vitally important strand in the rapid changes that are taking place. Primary care team organisation is variable and depends on several factors, e.g. organisational philosophy, local health care needs, constraints of professional organisations and expectations of powerful professional groups, team philosophies of care and individual motivation.

A useful way of understanding how relationships function within the primary care team is Anderson's (1969) three models of delegation, substitution and open access:

- *Delegation* is defined as the referral of a set of tasks by one professional group to another.
- *Substitution* describes a system where a paramedic sees the patient first with the doctor's mandate and support, which would be one of the functions of the nurse practitioner.
- *Open access* allows the patient to decide on the health professional most appropriate to deal with the problem. Implicit to the notion of open access is interdisciplinary teamwork.

These three models may all be present in a variety of ways in different primary care teams.

As a consequence of the NHS reforms and the increasingly mainstream feature of GP fundholding the frame of the team in primary health care is shifting rapidly. One of the tenets of the reforms was to decentralise decision making and to allow local diversity. This means that many different models of primary care organisation are emerging, from directly managed GP units to contracting community services from local Community Units or Trusts and primary health care nurses continuing to be employed by Trusts. There is debate about what constitutes the core and the extended team, which indicates perhaps an unhelpful preoccupation with structures and organisations, and is professionally driven rather than defining the team in relation to the patients' needs. Changing skill mix in primary care has resulted in some practice nurses and nurse practitioners becoming practice partners and other nurses working for the independent sector as providers. The relationship of this to skill mix and changing professional roles is explored in Chapter 7.

It is impossible to say what the effect of all this change will be. There are advantages and disadvantages to nurses of having GPs as managers and employers, as indeed there are to working within a hierarchical bureaucratic system. What is clear is that, despite all the past work that has examined teamwork in primary care, conclusions cannot be generalised to the present context. Perhaps we should take heed of Pearson and Jones' caution to avoid focusing on 'the rather nebulous concept of the primary health care team, but to replace it by an emphasis on cohesive multi-disciplinary working to achieve clearly established aims and objectives' (Pearson and Jones 1994: 1388).

Interprofessional education and training

Alongside the initiatives in collaborative working and teamwork in primary care has come the recognition that teamwork will not just happen by osmosis. There are two main approaches to learning interprofessionally, namely shared learning, which may mean a group of various professionals listening to the same lecture, and interactive or integrated learning, which entails mixed groups of students working together to solve problems.

There is evidence that most interprofessional education to date has been carried out at a post-qualifying level and, with the exception of a recent growth in masters courses (Storrie 1992), is of a short duration (CAIPE 1992). The majority of initiatives have not included medicine (CAIPE 1992). There is a view that models of good practice are learned through the socialisation of pre-qualifying education. Therefore the challenge of the 1990s is to explore new approaches to undergraduate and pre-qualifying education in medicine, nursing and other disciplines. This could be focused around important contemporary issues in primary care and, as Horder (1995) argues, should provide a common framework of knowedge, the breadth of which will bring new ways of solving patients' and clients' problems.

In view of the rapid changes in primary care there is an urgent need to provide relevant post-qualifying and continuing inter-professional education. On the whole, professional education has developed along separate discipline lines. This separation is influenced by historical divisions between the medical academic tradition based in Higher Education and nurse training determined by service requirements. This structural division is reinforced by different funding systems. Although the trend is now for nursing to move into Higher Education there are still differences in funding mechanisms and the way in which student numbers are determined. In terms of continuing education, the centrally negotiated scheme for general practitioners and the post-graduate training allowance allow them far greater flexibility and freedom. The continuing education of nurses working in primary care is subjected to various constraints depending on the context. Local service needs and funding affect the Health Authority-employed nurses, and the priorities of the individual GP employer influence whether or not, and how, practice nurses access training (Ross 1992, Killoran *et al.* 1993).

The current management view that individual professionals should be responsible for their own training should be interpreted in the light of the different funding systems for general practitioners and nurses. Having individual responsibility means that nurses are one step away from self-funding, whereas for general practitioners it means freedom of choice.

The structural difference between the two systems of education is a central problem in implementing innovative methods such as interprofessional training. The LOTS training is an example where interprofessional training has been possible and successful.

Conclusion

There are many developments in interprofessional work, evidenced by the recent plethora of literature and a journal dedicated to the topic. Primary health care is a pivotal part of the debate, providing opportunities for nursing to take part in leading change towards a user-centred and integrated service. There are many issues to resolve and further research to do, particularly into the effectiveness of teamwork related to patient outcomes.

Chapter 5
Quality of care

Summary

The influence of NHS reforms on quality of care and the consequent implications for nurses will be addressed in this chapter. The sometimes confusing and daunting terminology and definitions surrounding quality will be examined, together with the demands for measuring and evaluating practice. The contributions of nurses to quality initiatives and evaluation will be discussed.

Introduction

Assuring quality has become a major item on the policy agenda for change and has, over the past five years, been a focus of attention for professional organisations (Royal College of Nursing 1989, Royal College of General Practitioners 1985, Ross and Mackenzie 1991), for the Departments of Health (DoH 1989a) and for independent policy centres (Humphrey and Hughes 1992).

Within this context of political reform, decentralisation, together with the introduction of the internal market, has given impetus to the need to set standards and manage quality. A concern for quality is necessary to move towards a cost-effective and efficient service. Other influences that have evolved over the past 10 years, such as the need for self-regulation and improved performance by professionals, the recognition of greater accountability of professionals to society and user demand for more comprehensive health care and good service, are additional pressures for attention to quality (WHO 1989).

Quality in the context of NHS reforms

Managerialism

The changes in management policy initiated by the White Papers DoH 1989b and DoH 1989c see a turn around in the way in which the NHS is managed. It is a challenge to local management requiring the local sector, in the form of self-governing trusts and GP fundholders, to initiate the change themselves, rather than carrying out central government directives. The new model envisaged in the White Papers is that the centre sets the agenda for change as a framework for what is to be achieved. Then local units, GPs or community units, implement the change to meet local needs.

This is in contrast to previous NHS reforms where the centre has given strong direction as to how the change will be carried out, exerting influence through the various management tiers of a bureaucratic system. As Mitchell (1989) noted, one of the major challenges for success is whether or not local managers can initiate the reforms and whether or not the centre, in the form of the Management Executive, can give guidance rather than issue directives. The major difference in the present reforms is that the White Papers are about means not ends. Self-governing community trusts or GP units are the means of delivering a quality service to meet the needs of local communities at standards set locally (Mitchell 1989). The ends, such as improvement in patient care, equality of services, or consumer choice, are set out by central government, to be achieved by whatever means local management sees fit within available resources. The fear is that central government will not be able to resist continued directives and will scupper the aims of the reforms, as envisaged by author Sir Roy Griffiths (Best 1989). Analysis of government policy also points to difficulties for managers at local level who have to get used to a different model, one of greater autonomy and greater decision making, as they move towards being accountable for a more cost-effective service. The disadvantages of this model are that there may be loss of overall coherent planning and consequently short-term goals, raising questions as to whether or not it is possible to run the health service as a business. Few local nursing managers have been trained in commercial management and there have been some traumatic changes as a result of inept and insensitive local management, hampered by seemingly constant interference and contradictory advice from the Management Executive. As managers react to new demands, nurses have been at the receiving end of ill-thought-through ideas and have been frustrated by the lack of support for their own ideas about how practice might be improved.

Assuring quality then might be seen as a strategy for protecting the consumer on the one hand and professional practice on the other, in both cases by offering a counterbalance against the less desirable results of general management that demand cost effectiveness in a service that deals with health of people as the product. The Griffiths report defined general management as 'the responsibility, drawn together in one person, at different levels of the organisation, for planning implementation and control of performance' (DHSS 1983:11). This injection of managerialism into the NHS brings with it public accountability and has been strongly developed in primary care in the new role of GPs who are managerially accountable to the Family Health Services Authority. This managerialism seen at the interface of the GPs, Family Health Service Authorities (FHSAs) and community nursing will have a great impact on the primary care sector (Williams *et al.* 1993). The general practitioner is a linchpin in the reforms in primary health care, having fundholding responsibilities and being both a purchaser and a provider of care. Alongside this role come strong guidelines for improving responsiveness of services to consumer needs, giving consumers choice and increasing value for money and standards of care (NHSME 1991b).

The difficulties of applying general management principles in terms of quality have created problems that have led to concerns from practitioners about the aims of the NHS reforms. A content analysis of articles from nurses and their professional and union representatives in the *Nursing Times* from 1992 to 1993 reveals concerns about the reforms in terms of quality. Reducing quality of care for clients because of the difficulties of equating cost effectiveness and budgetary control with quality is a key issue. It is not only the radical change in thinking that is required, but also the speed of change and the lack of preparation that have led to some confusion and loss of morale among nurses in primary health care. Quality initiatives have often been developed in a piecemeal way across health districts. The directives from the Department of Health about quality have often been implemented without any operational planning or strategy, stifling the enthusiasm of clinical staff. A study from the Centre of Health Economics noted suspicions from staff about managers' motives in quality initiatives, confusion about what was expected of them and concerns that changes were more to do with meeting management goals than improving quality (Dalley *et al.* 1991).

Nursing influence on quality

The requirement for contracts between purchasers and providers to include statements about quality is, however, an opportunity to build in some control about what should be achieved and at what level.

It seems that there is a real opportunity for nurses to develop initiatives to improve primary health nursing (NHSME 1993a) when quality is central to the new reforms and nurses are explicitly encouraged or even directed to be involved in monitoring quality and effectiveness of health care (NHSME 1993b). Clear evidence of quality, linked with a demonstration of changed practice, is called for. Assuring quality involves all aspects of the reforms in areas where nurses have direct involvement and influence, such as user choice, cost effectiveness and better access to services. Certainly there is evidence from a survey of district Health Authorities in England and Wales (Dalley and Carr-Hill 1991) that nurses, who formed the largest group, almost a third, of all professionals surveyed, are responsive to the quality initiatives.

As well as being involved in clinical practice, nurses should, according to the Management Executive, play a role in the commissioning process, thus influencing policy by using their professional knowledge and skills to inform commissioners of the service. Four main areas are given:

- using epidemiological knowledge to assess health needs of populations and the impact of health interventions
- using communication skills to consult with individuals and groups about their health needs and feeding back decisions about health care to the community
- using experience from the clinical field to contribute to the negotiation of contracts and interpretation of clinical data that will inform them
- monitoring and evaluating services against contracts by drawing up measurable standards of care

(NHSME 1993b: 3.31–3.34)

Such involvement with the implementation of the reforms gives nurses in primary care central points of influence, all concerned with quality of care.

Salvage (1990) argues that nurses can exert key influence in the promotion of quality and suggests some key initiatives that will help to promote this role. One suggestion is for nurses 'to transform the nursing culture into one which constantly challenges established practice' (Salvage 1990:1), and this is discussed further in Chapter 7. The idea of having greater autonomy and independence is, however, one which equates well with greater influence on quality of care. The emphasis for Salvage is on meeting needs through individualised care. Nurses in primary health care should be able to exploit their position, which offers independence in practice on a day-to-day working basis. Added to this, primary health care has to be multi-disciplinary and intersectoral, if the reforms in community care are to be successful (DoH 1989c). Moving towards more control over quality of care cannot be achieved outside the context of reforms that emphasise effectiveness, efficiency and value for money.

It seems that there are five dimensions to be taken into account by primary health care nurses when striving towards assuring quality, as highlighted in Box 5.1.

Box 5.1 Dimensions to be taken into account when striving towards assuring quality

- the political issues of working within resource restraints and a contract culture
- the professional demands for nursing accountability and autonomy
- the centrality and sovereignty of the consumer
- the changing context of primary care where both health and social care are purchased and provided by a complex network of agencies
- the requirements for working in multi-disciplinary settings

---

Defining quality

Quality of care can be addressed at the individual level or inter-personal level, at the unit, organisational or local community political level, and at the government or national political level. These levels equate with what Rutgers and Berkel (1990) describe as the micro level, the meso level and the macro level.

Examining quality at a micro level (Redfern 1993) can be very valuable in informing nurses about their clinical practice, but in the current climate of change there is a need for primary health care nurses to be aware of external influences that impinge on and may restrict the quality of practice if not understood. This could, in turn, influence the definition of quality and the processes by which it may be assured.

One of the difficulties of addressing quality and understanding the processes has been demonstrated in the many definitions that abound. From the abundant international literature on the subject it now seems there is some sort of recognition that a specific definition of quality changes depending on whose perception is guiding the definition and at what level.

Changes in definition

There seems to be consensus that views of quality have changed over the years, from one of quality control, being just concerned with inspection-orientated one-off checks on a production line, to the current view of quality which is embodied in such terms as total quality management or continuous quality improvement (Kirk 1992, Redfern and Norman 1994). Davies (1992) notes these changes in Table 5.1.

Table 5.1 Changes in definition

	Traditional pre-1960	*Technocratic 1960s and 1970s*	*Total quality management (TQM) 1980s and 1990s*
Definition	La crème de la crème	Fitness for use Meeting requirements	A never-ending cycle of continuous improvement
Who defines quality?	Customers	Everybody knows what it is	Experts
Nature of quality		Product attribute	Process
What produces good quality		Good people and good materials	The right processes

Source: Amended from Davies 1992: 29

Quality through continuous improvement

Total quality management is 'a continuous striving, in "conversation" with the customer, towards an unattainable goal rather than an attainable product feature. Quality is a journey not a destination' (Davies 1992: 36).

After various false starts, this definition seems to be explicitly supported by the Management Executive and health units are providing published examples of how they have put this definition into practice through the recent Quality in Action initiative (NHSME undated a).

Some of the key reasons for change noted in the NHS reforms, such as need for more equal distribution of health care through equitable access, responding to client needs, higher expectations of a health care service and greater accountability to the public, are shared by other developed health care systems (Koch and Fairly 1993). Literature from the USA has influenced the development of quality processes in the NHS particularly at organisational level, where the implementation of quality being seen as a managed process is most evident.

The ideas for total quality management have been drawn from industry and in particular the Japanese car industry. Deming (1986) is the influential name that revolutionised the way in which quality was introduced into the car industry after the war. The concept of involving all levels of staff in assuring quality and the concept of managing quality as a process have influenced the understanding of quality assurance and management in the west and in the USA (Kirk 1992). Deming's main revolutionary idea, which has shifted quality measurement from the hands of the professional to the user, is that quality has meaning only in terms of the customer. Total quality management is a process by which quality can be managed. The emphasis is on managing rather than controlling (Oakland 1989). It has to be remembered, however, that much of the defining literature has been developed by working in institutional organisations.

Definitions at the level of the organisation become much more concerned with broad measurable outcomes such as those

of the joint Commission on Accreditation of Health Care Organ-
izations (JCAHO): 'the degree to which patient care services
increase the probability of desired patient outcomes and reduce
the probability of undesired outcomes, given the current state of
knowledge' (cited in Koch and Fairly 1993: 56). Koch and Fairly
(1993) note that today's quality approaches need a change in
management philosophy and organisational culture. The corporate
view is emphasised at the organisational level of achieving quality.
Synergy, the whole is more important than the parts, is integral to
total quality management. Each part of the system has an individual function, but all parts contribute to the aims and success of
the organisation. It is not just individuals doing their own thing,
but everyone working together.

Hierarchical or bureaucratic systems are not well placed for this
type of process. Nurses have been educated and socialised in a
bureaucratic culture, which engenders dependence on rituals and
routines, passivity towards authority and autocratic behaviour in
managers.The stability and rigidity that such a system engenders
do not promote the responsiveness and collaboration that total
quality management demands (Koch and Fairly 1993), hence
the need to change management philosophy and organisational
culture. The York study by Dalley and Carr-Hill (1991) notes that
components of total quality management match their findings very
closely. They stress the importance of management leadership
in engendering staff enthusiasm and establishing clear lines of
communication and a coherent strategy which has meaning for
both staff and management. Developing a culture for change is
emphasised, to ensure the reality and not just the rhetoric.

Difficulties of total quality management in primary health care

The commercial world has successfully empowered its customers
to define what they want and to become discerning about value
for money. Products are developed to meet customer demand
and audit measures the success of the product. In primary health

care the external customer, client, patient, or family require help from the practitioners in order to become more discerning and demanding in identifying their needs.

In terms of total quality management this is an essential part of the process of managing quality. Nurses who have the front line contact with external customers must therefore not only develop skills to carry out this educating and empowering process with external customers, but also be able to communicate their needs to other parts of the system. The success of a managed process of quality is reliant on both external and internal communication and requires a recognition that each department or unit is reliant on another for meeting external customer demands and ensuring quality. This network of internal customers, providing and purchasing a service within the organisation, is also integral to the process of managing quality (Masters and Schmele 1991). For instance, within a hospital the physiotherapy department provides a service for the wards in terms of promoting independence of patients, and the wards are purchasers of the service and reliant on it to assure standards of care are maintained. It is obvious that working in such an interdependent and co-operative way obliges staff to think and act differently (Arikian 1991). Although in institutions this is not an easy task, there are examples to show how it is being attempted and with some success (NHSME undated b).

One might say, however, that this approach to quality, developed within institutional organisations such as factories and hospitals, is not so easy to adopt in primary health care where units are disparate and difficult to define.

Total quality management may sound like another form of teamwork to nurses, a process that has been exhorted as the way forward in primary health care for many years (Royal Commission 1979) but has achieved only limited success (McClure 1984), certainly if measured in terms of improved patient outcomes. Few examples of total quality management are forthcoming from the Management Executive in terms of primary health, particularly if extended to the whole gamut of co-operation across social and health services.

User influence on quality

Perhaps the way forward is to conceptualise quality not just in terms of a managed process, a system by which quality can be assured or guaranteed, but to concentrate on quality as being influenced by the user more than by the professional. It is this aspect of total quality management that seems to have the most potential for ensuring quality in primary care, rather than the emphasis on the process of managing quality on an institution wide basis. Perhaps a corruption of McCaffery's (1983) definition of pain would be an appropriate slogan: 'quality is what the patient or client says it is'. This, of course, means an even more flexible system of management, but perhaps one that is easier to implement in primary care. After all, attempts at meeting the needs of the patient or client, the external customer, are not new in primary health even if the terminology changes. The process by which the patient or client might be included in decisions in the primary health care team is, however, very new. Although the concept has been discussed from an epidemiological perspective (Anderson 1969), drawing on social work practice (Webb and Hobdell 1980) and draws from district nursing (Ross 1980), application is perhaps the greatest challenge for professionals working in the community. Interprofessional work is discussed in more detail in Chapter 4.

The difficulties of professionals working together are well described by Webb and Hobdell (1980) and 15 years later their observations are very relevant to the current NHS reforms in which groups of professionals are to draw up programmes of care to meet health needs, social needs or both. The importance of patient sovereignty is noted as one way in which the competing status of the different professionals can be abated. By recognising patient or client needs as paramount in the decision-making process, it is argued that the authority to make decisions about patients' or clients' needs based on professional knowledge will be of less significance and this will lead to less professional rivalry and struggle for power. Contribution to decision making about health care 'must arise from the possession of knowledge relevant to the client's own feelings of well-being, not from the possession of a particular body of theoretical knowledge' (Webb and Hobdell 1980:107). This is described as the authority of relevance in contrast to the authority of knowledge used to legitimatise professional decisions. This principle can be applied to the implementation of quality, to the process of managing quality and to the setting of standards and evaluation. A further extension of this discussion is that frequently those with little authority of knowledge are closest to the client, patient or family. For instance, nurses may be closer than doctors, home helpers may be closer than social workers, or support workers may be closer than nurses. Adhering to the principle of the authority of relevance will become a complex process as more unqualified staff are employed and come to see themselves as patient advocates.

Changes in management culture and philosophy (Katz and Green 1992) must impinge on the way in which professionals perceive their power over each other and over the patient or client. The identification of external customers includes patients and clients, their relatives, and the local community, and is the starting point for meeting individual health needs.

An example of this changing culture is illustrated by nurses working with mothers in the community as a *Health of the Nation* initiative, developed in Dublin and known as the Community Mothers' Programme (Lloyd 1993). It was piloted in 1983 by the Eastern Health Board in Dublin. Families from disadvantaged areas were visited monthly by public health nurses – who in Ireland do the work of district nurses, health visitors and midwives – to focus on nutrition, health care and development, aiming to avoid crisis intervention. Evaluation was a part of this project and showed positive effects on parenting skills. This project was extended to involve the mothers themselves, who were recruited to support first- and second-time parents with infants under 1 year. The community mothers are experienced mothers who have a willingness to contribute to the community, are friendly and literate and are recommended by other professionals. They visit

parents in their own home for one hour, once a month by appointment, facilitate mother and toddler groups, arrange speakers and
work with travelling families. The programme discriminates in
favour of disadvantaged areas in a part of Ireland where there is
70 per cent unemployment and social problems such as alco-
holism, child abuse, violence and depression are high. Assuring
quality in this programme is not just the prerogative of professionals; mothers themselves are experts. The continued evaluation
of such projects will be important and can be addressed not just
in terms of *Health of the Nation* targets, but also in terms of cost
and benefit to the first, second-time and community mothers, and
of an assessment of cost benefit.

Identifying internal customers is, however, a very much
more hazardous process. For instance, a similar example to
the one previously described for a hospital setting, the promotion
of independence in elderly people, could include district nurses,
general practice nurses, health visitors, occupational therapists,
physiotherapists, home helps, support workers, doctors and
voluntary workers. Even if we can assume that the original core
primary health care team of nurses and GPs are able to work
together, others in the team may be employed and funded by
different agencies, and since the new directives that arise from
The NHS and Community Care Act (DoH 1990b) emphasise a
separation of health and social care, we can see the complexities
of defining, let alone evaluating, quality of care.

Specialisation in nursing in primary care settings may also
make it more difficult to gain a corporate image, or shared goals
for quality, requiring negotiation skills across clinical specialities.
The move by nurses to identify their own special contributions
to the team, as a reaction against the perceived merging of roles
by the UKCC (1991) on the one hand and the need to identify
nurses' contribution towards health gain in the face of efficiency
measures on the other, increases boundaries and makes the
chances of achieving shared philosophies towards quality
more difficult. Cost-effectiveness measures, resulting in reduced
numbers of qualified community nurses, may well force spurious

specialisation in an attempt to defend roles and jobs. This will not encourage the sort of co-operation required for team working.

A review of definitions

The purpose here is not to be pessimistic about achieving quality care by nurses in primary care, but merely to demonstrate that guidance or stated 'ends' from the NHS Management Executive about quality will need to consider the contexts and not assume that it is possible for all initiatives to follow examples set in institutions, in health centres or in GP practices that might be regarded as independent units or organisations. The hope that the local units will be able to decide their own means by which they are to achieve high-quality care for a community has to be realised. Certainly too much direction here will thwart any attempts to be innovative in achieving quality outcomes in the interdependent areas of health and social care. While examples of quality initiatives may be motivating, they may also be daunting to practitioners and may engender excessive competitiveness. Also, other developments in policy must be taken into account, if the aims of achieving high quality within given resources are to be realised. Total quality management is in danger of moving from managing the process of quality to merely measuring outcomes if we place too much emphasis on definitions similar to that of the JCAHO (1990).

Redfern (1993) argues that quality is a personal and esoteric concept. 'We want to pin it down but in doing so we may lose the magic of the elusive ray of light in our search for concreteness' (Redfern 1993:141). This paper analyses definitions of health care and notes the difficulties of defining quality in terms of outcomes for patient or client, the individual who is in a unique position regarding health status. As Redfern points out, patients 'may not know what they require, may know what they want but be unable to articulate it, or may want something known to be harmful' (Redfern 1993:142). Added to this might be that what they want is not attainable.

In this type of definition the impetus for assessing quality depends on negotiated outcomes. At an individual level this may well be achieved if the outcome is fairly broad. Such goals as ensuring dignity, reducing pain, or promoting self-esteem can be achieved in different ways and are subjectively measured by each patient or client. This is in contrast to looking at outcomes on a production line, where the emphasis on increasing quality is to improve the quality of the work area through greater motivation and job satisfaction. On the factory floor a satisfied worker improves quality, but the variables that influence quality with patients will be more than job satisfaction and technical competence, and will include interpersonal skills and recognition of personal needs.

The views put forward by Luthert and Robinson (1993) also recognise the difficulties of defining quality and its elusive nature, but suggest that the term assurance alongside quality requires some type of guarantee of quality, and therefore a clear level of achievement has to be set.

Evaluating and measuring quality

Assuring quality, by whatever means appropriate, includes measurement, evaluation and, most importantly, change. Unless this cyclical process is maintained, the dynamic process will be compromised (Norman and Redfern 1990). The point is made that measuring quality is about identifying agreed expectations in the form of standards or goals, comparing what is happening in practice against these pre-set standards and making changes to practice to meet the pre-set standards. This is a simple and clear process of assuring quality through measurement. One has to be careful, however, that change is not made for the sake of it, and, if standards are being met, good practice can be identified and maintained. Furthermore, the result of evaluation may be to change the standards or goals rather than the practice. At this early stage of nurses' experience in setting standards, it may be that the goals set are too stringent or unattainable. There has to be the confidence to accept that standards are not always perfect.

It is clear, however, that standards of practice must be achievable, observable, desirable and measurable (Royal College of Nursing 1989). This bottom-up approach, developed by Kitson (1986) and based on the structure, process, outcome framework of Donabedian (1966), is one that has had great influence in the UK. A synthesis of the work of Donabedian (1966) and Wilson (1987) has guided the development of standards of care at the Royal Marsden Hospital, showing how research and attention to quality can be brought together to guide practice (Luthert and Robinson 1993). There is certainly enough literature on assuring quality (Luthert and Robinson 1993, Redfern 1993, Kitson 1987) for nurses to begin to develop and refine what is mainly institutionally-based work and to apply it to primary health care.

Standards and guidelines for practice

Much literature has also been written on how to write standards. The difficulty for nurses is that the intricacies and minutiae of defining the standard may detract from the overall rationale of assuring quality of care. One of the major problems in setting standards is where to begin or on which area of practice to focus.

A desirable starting point for standard setting in primary health care is assessment of need at either an individual or a local level. Epidemiological data provides nurses with a profile of the local community within which individuals and family groups live their lives. This level of information can be interpreted in the light of information from other sources. For instance, we know from consumer groups and research that there are common needs for disabled, such as improved access, aids for the home, help at times that are appropriate, support for carers and respite for families; but the identification of numbers of disabled people *per se* is not enough. An individual focus for that particular client group in that particular locality has to be given. As information systems become more sophisticated, data from local councils, public health departments, voluntary groups and individual patient records can be integrated to form a comprehensive and accessible database, which is available for making decisions about standards of quality (McNaught 1991).

Standards then will be set at various levels, national or local, for various purposes, for purchasing or providing, and their specificity will vary accordingly. National targets have been published for reduction of death rates from coronary heart disease by at least 40 per cent by the year 2000 (DoH 1992). Carers' groups would also like to see national standards set for the processes of assessment of elderly people before drawing up a package of care under the Community Care Act (further discussed in Chapter 6).

The contributions of nurses to such targets could be detailed at local level and carried out at local clinics or community centres or between hospital and community units, as shown in the Good Heart project initiated by health visitors in Chester (Evans 1994). At this level the process criteria of intervention for a rehabilitation programme will become specific, and involve a range of professionals working between secondary and primary care (Evans 1994). It is not difficult to see how levels of outcomes vary from the broad indicators of health at national level, such as incidence of coronary heart disease, to the more specific outcomes in terms of changed health behaviour. Audit can be used to compare present practice with changes in practice following intervention by looking at both process and outcome criteria and thus evaluating effectiveness and, if possible, efficiency.

The national standards have given some focus and it may be very appropriate for nurses to demonstrate their contributions. Such targets will also be used in contracts. This type of work has been ongoing in Trent, where comprehensive guidelines to reduce the morbidity of asthma have been drawn up for contracting, particularly in relation to primary health care (Trent Health 1993). These guidelines, drawn up by a multi-disciplinary group, are informative and clear and give insight into the contracting process. Both national targets (DoH 1992) and local contracts are likely to have a strong influence on audit and standard setting.

It is also hoped, however, that this government's acknowledgement of the importance of health promotion (DoH 1992) will be used as a framework for standards that may be more appropriate to some individual needs. Rehabilitation and tertiary prevention are common requisites in primary health, but outcomes are less easy to measure (Barriball and Mackenzie 1993). They may require long-term multi-disciplinary interventions to be effective and are therefore less cost effective in the short term, and may be less popular on the contracting agenda when there are many other areas that demonstrate achievement.

Primary health care nurses do not come to standard setting without some knowledge of what happens in patient situations, nor some knowledge of the local scene and pattern of health needs, nor without some concerns about care. Audit of frequent activities, such as assessments in district nursing, counselling in psychiatric nursing and advising mothers on infant feeding, might also provide a starting point for setting standards and giving guidance to practice.

The setting of criteria against which to measure the process or the outcome may well be drawn from research-based knowledge (Luthert and Robinson 1993) and could help to prioritise some of the activities for the primary health care team. Interventions that have been shown to be ineffective, such as routine screening of children, would at least be discarded, and those interventions where there is good research to guide practice, such as leg ulcer prevention or health education for specific groups, could be used to establish measurable criteria.

Using profiles of caseload and practice, together with knowledge of treatment and prevention of leg ulcers, and an audit of assessment, McCready (1995) showed that district nurses needed guidance. Protocols were established and standards drawn up, and after one year a second audit showed a reduction from 9 per cent to 8 per cent (n = 126) in the number of patients with leg ulceration. Taking into account that the average cost of treating one patient each year is £670, this project demonstrates the use of the dynamic process of quality assurance, starting with audit, through standard setting to changed practice and subsequently measurement of effectiveness.

Standard setting may become sterile and theoretical, frustrating and time consuming, if not carried out with a good helping of common sense and willingness to compromise, in order to get to a starting point that is subsequently linked to guidelines for practice. Conventionally written standards detail a level of performance and state criteria for measurement in terms of process, what should be done, and outcomes, changes in clients' health status or behaviour. Details of structure, such as records of health needs, staff education, accommodation and facilities, relate to a number of process and outcome criteria, but, once reconciled with resources, do not need to be included in every standard statement. Audit of processes or assessment of health needs by population assessment, or a combination of both, can be used as the starting point for standards and practice or clinical guidelines.

Whether or not the standard setting is at national or local level, there is no doubt that outcome is the most important point of measurement in the NHS reforms. One would hope that such outcomes are not just about cost effectiveness, but also reflect some of the other dimensions of quality described by Maxwell (1984), such as access to services, relevance to need at community level, effectiveness for individual patients, equity or fairness and social acceptability.

As Bloch has noted, the type of evaluation that links the process, what the professional does, to the outcome, in terms of patient benefits, is the ultimate goal of medical and nursing care (Bloch 1975). Twenty years on this is still the focus of attention in health care evaluation. It is now complicated by the fact that nurses are required to demonstrate their value to health care provision (Bond and Thomas 1991).

Multi-disciplinary evaluation and clinical audit

Measuring outcomes in primary health is not the prerogative of one professional group. From the patients' or clients' points of view, it is important that the service results in good care, whoever provides it. For the providers it may be important to determine what constitutes good care and who delivers it, in order that it can be repeated or amended. For the purchaser a broader measure which results in hard statistical data may be needed. The primary health care team will need to decide if they are evaluating the service as a whole, including such elements as patient satisfaction with discharge or waiting times, or if they are measuring change in clients' behaviour or health status, as demonstrated by improved knowledge of risk factors in heart disease or improved mobility following a stroke. As research has shown, detailing and linking the process and outcome of care is difficult enough (Bond and Thomas 1992), but separating nursing interventions from other interventions, lay and professional, is even more difficult (Redfern 1993, Kitson 1987).

Taking into account the importance of reliability and validity, process and outcome congruence, and feasibility and practicality of outcome measurement (Shaw 1984), it is not surprising that some authorities suggest more research needs to be carried out to provide appropriate measures. In the absence of perfect answers, however, perhaps the best that can be said is that, where possible, appropriate existing measures should be used (Bond and Thomas 1992). In this respect we have a choice of generic measures, Monitor being widely used (Dalley and Carr-Hill 1991), or of specific measures, such as the Barthel index used for activities of daily living, or a combination of specific measures that attempt to measure more than just physical improvement. Reviews of measuring instruments help professionals to make decisions from a plethora of literature (Harvey 1991, Wilkin *et al.* 1992).

It is recognised that outcome measurement is in its infancy and that a sharing of ideas will improve our knowledge (UK Clearing House 1993). While GPs have taken the lead in audit in primary health (Irvine and Irvine 1991), the move towards multi-disciplinary audit is welcome and necessary, given that no single approach to audit will suit every circumstance (Humphrey and Hughes 1992). Although we have information on nursing audit

(NHSME undated c) as part of the process for evaluating health care and measuring standards, some of which information has been confusing to say the least, we have little information on what measures to use or how to select them. More recently, the Department of Health has emphasised that clinical audit is not just to be regarded as medical audit, but should be 'undertaken by multi-professional health care teams, focused on the patient and developed in a culture of continuing evaluation and improvement of clinical effectiveness, focusing on patient outcomes' (NHSME undated d). It is a welcome move and hopefully the money made available for audit projects will result in good evaluations of such practice.

Establishing multi-disciplinary audit has been the focus of primary health care teams in various parts of the country in an effort to identify topics for team audit. The difficulties of multi-disciplinary audit as well as the positive effects on quality were raised. The common findings are that effective audit is linked to improved quality of care and influenced by good teamwork (Hearnshaw in press).

Conclusion

Assuring quality is an integral part of the NHS reforms and it is clear from policy and research literature that nurses are one of the major professional groups to be involved in these policy initiatives. The success in channelling this motivation and enthusiasm lies with managers at all levels, but particularly at unit level. Increasingly, in the community, appointments with a quality remit are being made at a clinical level. The development of special posts, such as nurse advisers in quality assurance, may have helped to promote the first initiatives, although some see that as merely a result of the introduction of general management and the horizontal promotion of senior nurses in the reorganisation of senior management structures.

As in other aspects of the NHS reforms, the paperwork and rhetoric that accompany the implementation seem to supersede the goal. All nurses, however, want to improve quality of health care. To achieve this Dalley and Carr-Hill suggest

> that the enthusiasm at the front-line for a wide variety of quality activities be knitted together with management's leadership and strategic thinking – within the framework of a corporate strategy. The current catch phrase "management led, bottom fed" seems to capture the spirit of the approach very well.
>
> (Dalley and Carr-Hill 1991: 21)

In primary health, where teamwork and intersectoral working are essential, it may seem that such suggestions will result in too bureaucratic an approach. Each unit will have to work out its own strategy, where the professionals at the clinical level will have influence over the strategy.

Total quality management is not the panacea for ensuring quality. The most important aspect of the principles is that the organisation should offer primary health care nurses the chance to bring about change. New management structures in themselves do not necessarily mean that quality of care is given (Hughes 1990). Nurses themselves have the responsibility to work in ways which promote good quality care. Some characteristics of good practice have resulted from a recent study using 122 clinical experts (Butterworth 1994) and are similar to those recognised by other professional organisations in primary health care (Mackenzie 1989). Resulting guidelines require managers and primary health care nurses to work in ways that will produce good quality care.

Of equal or perhaps more importance for nurses is the interface with general practitioners and other agencies in primary health care. Here we have very little understanding, let alone guidelines, for quality initiatives, and it is here that primary health care nurses will be the pioneers of quality. They should not be daunted by the inconsistent terminology that surrounds quality assurance, or some of the confusing guidelines issued by the centre. Waiting for clear definitions will only delay good ideas and encourage sterile academic argument. Primary health care nurses have enough expertise to contribute to the debate from a clinical level by engaging with policy makers and full-time researchers to enhance practice.

Chapter 6
Family carers

Summary

This chapter will examine the role of carers in looking after dependent family members. It will consider why this phenomenon is so high on the policy agenda and how the nurse in primary health care might use the knowledge from research to enhance the caring role of the family, while at the same time resisting the drive to give the family a responsibility it is not able to fulfil. Although there are a substantial number of children who act as carers, this chapter will concentrate on adult carers, those over 16 years of age. Given the demographic trends and the fact that the peak age for caring occurs in the adult range (OPCS 1992), it is expected that the majority of caring activities in the community will be centred on this group.

The term carer is the terminology used here to describe someone other than professionals or organised volunteers, 'who regularly helps a relative or friend who is disabled or ill, with tasks like dressing, shopping or household tasks, or who offers sorts of practical or emotional support' (Robinson and Yee 1991: 116). The terms informal carer and primary carer will be used with reference to particular literature.

Contribution of carers to community care

Graham, in her clear exposition of informal care in the community, summarises the features of informal care as embracing 'a broad category of care which is unpaid and home based and governed by the moral and emotional ties of kinship' (Graham 1991: 508), normally relating to dependants with long-term health problems, many of whom might otherwise be institutionalised. Such features present difficulties for those involved and challenges for nurses, who are part of this pluralistic pattern of care and who often work at the interface between carers and the other sectors offering health and social care.

The shifting emphasis from 'care in the community' to 'care by the community' was quite clearly stated in the government White Paper entitled *Growing Older* (DHSS 1981a). Subsequently, community care reforms (DoH 1989c) have further emphasised that 'the great bulk of community care is provided by friends, family and neighbours' (para. 1.9) and that this group should be clearly identified as forming part of a diverse pattern of care including the statutory, independent and voluntary sectors as well as carers. Indeed, money from central government was transferred to Local Authorities when the Community Care Act came into force in 1993. This money is to be spent on maintaining people in their own homes rather than transferring them to residential homes. It was also clearly stated that carers should be involved in the assessment and the development of the care planned during the process of defining a care package (DoH 1989c).

Help from groups, family, neighbours and friends has been promoted by both Labour and Conservative governments as part of the drive towards family responsibility. While no doubt for many people caring for dependent relatives in the family home is the preferred option, it is also cost effective for government since the carers are unpaid. In 1985 the Audit Commission calculated that carers saved the government over £3,000 a year per elderly person cared for, and concluded that 'carers have needs and rights – since their work is important to the economy of the health and social services' (Audit Commission 1985: 43). This recognition of the contribution of carers to the health and social care of the elderly in economic terms does not acknowledge the social, physical and emotional personal costs to carers.

The General Household Survey (GHS) (Green 1988) estimated that the numbers of people caring for others who live in the community was 6 million. The size of the problem that this figure

revealed gave new impetus to the carers' lobby and in particular the campaigns of carers' organisations (Carers' National
Association 1992), who were not slow to point out that a requirement of the new community care policy is for health and social
services authorities to consult carers when assessing the needs
of disabled and elderly people in the local populations. The GHS
has for the first time drawn attention to the large number of
people who have caring responsibilities and who themselves have
health and social needs. The fact that the topic of caring was
included in the 1985 General Household Survey at the request
of the Departments of Health and Social Security is more
evidence that carers are now part of the policy agenda.

The interest in carers and the high profile they have achieved
since the early 1980s is mainly due to the feminist movement and
related research about the role of women in the home, and to the
articulate and politically aware interest groups who have lobbied
on behalf of carers. This is not to say that the plight of carers is
any better than it was 10 years ago, only that it has been brought
to the attention of government, public and professionals.

Ambiguities and inequalities in services to carers

The emphasis on family obligation by the New Right is likely
to lead to ambiguity in service provision, on the one hand
offering support to carers as encouragement to continue their
informal care, but on the other withholding services that may
encourage carers to withdraw from caring for their relatives.

Gender

While the feminist literature has concentrated on the plight of
women in caring, the GHS showed that men also carry out caring
responsibilities and that the proportions of men and women
are not markedly different. The 1990 GHS (OPCS 1992) noted
a rise in the total number of carers to 16.8 million and showed a

greater number of men involved in caring (13 per cent of adult
men as opposed to 16 per cent of adult women) than had previously
been described.

The secondary analysis of General Household Surveys (Arber
and Gilbert 1993) dispels some of the myths engendered by feminist research that the majority of carers are women and that
women carers are less likely to get help from statutory and voluntary sources than men. According to this analysis, the amount
of services seems to be based on the type of household in which
the dependent person lives, rather than on the gender of the carer.
Where elderly and 'severely disabled' people are living together
as spouses, caring is shared almost equally between wives
and husbands. Indeed, where the relationship is one that has
been built up over years, e.g. spouses or unmarried daughters
living with their mother, then the role of carer is taken on as
part of the relationship, a gradual move from interdependency
to dependency, as age or disease renders one member to become
dependent. In the situation where the dependent elderly family
member has to move into another household for care, however,
the carer is most likely to be a married woman and not a man.
This is where the gender inequality in care is most likely to be
seen (Arber and Gilbert 1993). For instance, district nurses are
less likely to visit or carry out a full range of tasks in households
where there is a married daughter. The overall conclusion,
however, is that

> the major source of variation in the amount of support
> services received by elderly infirm men and women seems
> to be not the gender of the recipients or the gender of the
> carer, but the kind of household in which they live and, in
> particular, where there are others in the household who
> could take on the burden of caring.
>
> (Arber and Gilbert 1993: 141)

To some extent this is also noted by Parker and Lawton (1991)
in their analysis of the General Household Survey, where they

were able neither to prove nor disprove arguments about bias in service provision in favour of those with male carers.

This type of analysis is of great help when planning the services to those who are disabled and to their carers. Professional services may make assumptions about the ability or willingness of married women and their families to cope with ageing and increasingly dependent relatives. The point is made that in other relationships of caring, such as parents looking after children, the majority of children will grow up and become independent. The caring role is therefore fairly predictable and planned for. In the case of spouses and of single children living with parents the dependency develops gradually, is not unexpected and can be planned for to some extent. In the case of elderly dependent kin moving into an already established household, however, the responsibilities of caring may be very disruptive. It is not that caring is any less arduous for the spouse or the unmarried child, but that the whole family must come to terms with the new situation.

Further analysis of the GHS survey (Parker and Lawton 1994) also demonstrates that some disabled and older people live relatively independent lives using a combination of services such as appropriate housing or adaptations and therefore need only minimal support from family or friends. So while the figures show the numbers of people who say they receive support, for some it may be very little, and indeed good assessment of dependency and provision of appropriate equipment and housing may reduce the numbers of carers. It also appears that there is an increasing difference in the involvement of carers between those who are heavily involved, particularly with very old and mentally impaired relatives, and those who are helping relatives or friends who can live alone if supported by appropriate housing and other facilities. As Parker and Lawton (1994) note, this has implications for policy.

At a local level assessments should be able to differentiate and to identify a focus for services, thus making better use of resources. If appropriate and acceptable equipment can be made available, then district nurses, for instance, can use their resources to support other carers who have greater involvement and who need more help, rather than keep people on the caseload unnecessarily (Badger *et al.* 1989). This will need good evaluation of local services, such as that carried out by Ross and Campbell (1992). In this study it was clearly shown that not only were some aids and equipment inappropriate for disabled people, but also delivery took far too long. Indeed, in some instances, two district nurses have been required to visit a home to lift and care for patients because the lifting hoist or other equipment was not suitable or acceptable. Close working between all sectors in the Local Authority and nurses in primary health care is required if the Community Care Act is to work successfully for carers.

Ethnic and minority groups

In analysing the research literature it seems that fairly arbitrary reasons are used for providing services. Those who cope well, or are perceived as having abilities to cope, are obliged to do so and offered very little help. Assumptions are also made about black and Chinese populations. Their needs are often overlooked due to myths that black and ethnic minority communities living in the UK have well-established kinship groups (Gunaratnum 1993) and that they are mainly young and mobile (Baxter 1988). It is obvious from those who work with such communities that there are old and disabled family members living here. The OPCS survey (1988) found that there were no significant differences in the prevalence of disability between adults in West Indian and Asian households and those of the white population.

Apart from Asian populations from the Indian subcontinent and Afro-Caribbean communities, the Chinese community is the third largest ethnic minority group in Britain, having increased dramatically with the emigration of families from Hong Kong (Au *et al.* 1992). Family and filial obligations are traditionally strong in Chinese populations (Mackenzie and Holroyd in press). There are, however, other factors that also contribute to the poor uptake of services by the Chinese in Britain: the majority do not speak English; they are unwilling to seek help outside the family; they work long unsocial hours; populations are dispersed and small and go unnoticed (Au *et al.* 1992). Indeed, uptake of services is an unreliable indicator of need as many of the services are inaccessible, due to lack of information, and inappropriate, due to lack of understanding or insensitivity towards cultural values. It is feared that the situation will worsen as the current concentration on cost effectiveness favours large-scale provision and ignores smaller groups with particular needs (Gunaratnam 1993).

Accessing the services

Whatever the group the accessibility of the service needs to be addressed. Frequently carers will have access to the service only indirectly through the referral of the dependant. It seems that legitimate access to the service for carers in their own right as consumers is difficult and frequently linked to the needs of the client (Twigg and Atkin 1994). Despite the exhortations to involve users (Carers' National Association undated a) by giving information and publishing services, carers are in a particularly difficult position. Once they become involved in care it is demanding and time consuming, and leaves little energy for anything else.

Assessing carers' needs

Those services, such as district nurses (Atkinson 1992) and community psychiatric nurses (Keady and Nolan 1994), that are most frequently involved with carers of dependent adults are in a key position to assess carers' needs. Such assessment should ideally start before discharge from hospital, although discharge planning is notoriously poor, as described in Chapter 1. This is a time of high stress for family members who might be expected to take on the responsibility for a frail or dependent relative. A comprehensive assessment of need should be carried out to identify which patients have willing carers and needs that can be provided for in the home, and which need alternative provision (Nolan and Grant 1992). The most important function that nurses have is to ensure that carers are able to make informed decisions about their role and that they are not obliged to take the responsibility just because the hospital consultant deems it appropriate. Assessments are often made just about functional performance and hence ability to cope with physical tasks, although it is the emotional and psycho-social factors in caring for dependent relatives that are often the most burdensome (Lewis and Meredith 1988), sometimes leading to a breakdown in relationship, yet largely ignored in discharge planning (Nolan and Grant 1992). Nurses in primary health are in a position to provide invaluable information about the difficulties of family support and may alert hospital staff to the needs of carers so that appropriate preparations can be made and impossible situations avoided (Newman 1991).

It is generally agreed that care giving results in burden or stress and much research has been carried out to identify precise measures of this construct, particularly in the area of mental health (Vitaliano *et al.* 1991). Burden scales have the potential to help in the measurement of individual assessments before and after discharge. The difficulties of describing the concept precisely, however, have made it impossible to draw conclusions from research that often gives conflicting results (Braithwaite 1992). The plethora of burden scales has caused Zarit (1989) to question the need for further research studies into stress and burden and to recommend more emphasis upon the evaluation of community programmes and upon closer working between researchers and practitioners. Indeed, it might be said that research on carer burden should be related more closely to the realities of practice. Scales to help professionals and carers assess and articulate the dimensions of burden constitute a move towards putting the vast array of burden and stress research to more practical use (Novak and Guest 1989, Robinson 1983, Kosberg and Cairl 1986), and towards recognising that, despite generalisations, burden is directly related to context and must be assessed in context (Braithwaite 1992).

For nurses the identification of carers in the population is the first step in assessing carers' needs and interests. A case-finding approach is described by a district nurse in Kettering (Mawby 1993) who used the practice records to identify the needs of carers previously unknown to the district nurse. This assessment of the practice population resulted in discussion with the carers about their needs and in the subsequent establishment of a carers' support group and shows the importance of case-finding. The Carers' National Association (undated b) is also encouraging carers themselves to ask for an assessment of their dependent relatives, giving clear explanation of provision under the new reforms and an example of an assessment form. Examples of involving carers also come from Nottingham (Adcock 1991) and Sutton (Ramdas 1991). Assessment of carers' needs inevitably leads to the question of whether or not carers have a choice in taking on their caring role.

Carer choice

The question of carer choice is one of the contradictions of a policy that promotes care by the community on the one hand and client choice on the other. This dilemma is highlighted in the White Paper on community care:

> The decision to take on a caring role is never an easy one. However, many people make that choice and it is right that they should be able to play their part in looking after those close to them. But it must be recognised that carers need help and support if they are to continue to carry out that role.
>
> (DoH 1989c: para 1.9)

The White Paper goes on to emphasise 'assisting people to live independent lives in their own homes and avoiding unnecessary institutional care'.

Here we see part of the dilemma for carers. It is implied in this statement that carers and families have a choice, but it is only a choice if they wish to look after their relatives at home. If they do not wish or are unable to look after their relatives, they are still going to be encouraged to do so by agencies and professionals in order to avoid unnecessary institutionalisation. Hence meeting carers' needs is a very complex issue.

A further question in provision of services is whether or not carers, having entered the political agenda, are to be regarded as consumers and users of the service or as providers. The National Association of Health Authorities (1993) notes that the new models of health based on substitution place more responsibility on families for long-term care with little option for refusal. Substitution of home for institutional care means that relatives are expected to take patients back into the home with more complex health problems and with less opportunity for long-term institutionalised care. In this situation, therefore, they are providers. Taking this argument to one extreme it could be said that treating carers as providers and paying them for services could enhance their care giving, as well as meet their need for financial help.

Ungerson (1993) makes the point that the private domain of the home in which caring is carried out makes it more difficult for decisions to be made about rights that are associated with citizenship and are part of the public domain. Caring is carried out within a relationship frequently based on love and obligation and may not be amenable to the intervention of the State in terms of how often or what type of care dependent relatives should receive as of right from their family. For instance, the rights of the carer and the dependant may be different and difficult to reconcile. Care based on an employment contract, in which the carer gets paid for services rendered, may well change the nature of the relationship and the expectations of the dependant. Some dependants, however, may be getting second-class care simply by virtue of the fact that their carers are equally infirm. In such cases a contract would not enhance the care but might highlight areas of deficit or need.

The unpredictability of disabling conditions sometimes causes difficulties as to whether or not carers should receive paid leave from employment in order to look after people experiencing more acute phases of disability. For those in the process of caring this is an academic argument, but for those in the planning of services such considerations underline the need for more flexibility in the service and in the assessment process.

Offering flexibility of service

Flexibility in the service is the key word in the arguments of those who champion the cause of disabled people (Oliver 1988). Demedicalisation of disability is called for and a recognition that disability and the resulting handicap are socially constructed and therefore require intersectoral co-operation in primary health care. Oliver is outrightly critical of the community nursing team, particularly the district nurse, whom he perceives to be more concerned with medical tasks than with the maintenance care of those with a disability. He states that district nurses conceptualise disability as a medical problem, not a social problem, and treat people with disabilities in a paternalistic manner, as patients not users. Carers in these situations are expected to cope or to find other alternatives for help. Certainly the community nursing service, in the case described by Oliver, was not able to meet the carer's demands for someone to help wash and dress a young man in time to go to work. Indeed, some district nurses would agree with this analysis and would hope that since this paper was written the situation has been improved by changes in education, the drive towards new practitioner roles, discussed in Chapter 7, and the new community structures.

Offering flexibility through respite care within the home is one option that has been taken up by a team in Preston. This service, co-ordinated by district nurses, utilises the services of nursing auxiliaries and a registered nurse, who carry out activities in the home to allow the carer to have time out. Liaison with other agencies also helps to expand the service (Wilson and

Bannister 1989). This type of initiative provides an alternative to institutional respite care, which is not always acceptable to the dependent person or the carer.

In some instances, changes in policy have merely compounded the difficulties of offering flexibility in the services by separating out social and health care responsibilities. Caseload management for district nurses has become more difficult because of the fragmentation of care between different agencies. Similarly the purchaser/provider split, where policy suggests that nurses are expected to be more of a provider than a purchaser, does not meet the reality of practice, where in fact nurses are required to use the skills of both providing and purchasing services for patients.

If packages of care are developed as envisaged in the policy arrangements, then flexible provision could be implemented. It seems, however, that although nurses are extensively involved in case management and with people who have long-term health problems, there is little assessment of carers' needs (Bergen 1994). This might seem surprising, given the extensive literature on the subject and the recent policy initiatives, but such schemes are still in their infancy and are not without difficulties, although tentative gains for carers are described by the Darlington Community Care Project (Challis *et al*. 1989). Learning to work across agencies and finding the time required to co-ordinate care (Bergen 1994), together with increasing demands on carers (Twigg *et al*. 1990), means that this type of interagency working, which could be so beneficial for carers, has yet to develop fully.

Partnership with carers

Assumptions are made that partnership with clients and carers is a good thing. This is supported by policy and the pervading ideologies of self-care in nursing (Orem 1991).

Consumerism in health implies patient or client participation in making decisions about personal health or about health care. Brearley (1990) sees the user as a client or patient, or member of the client's or patient's family. As such the carer may be a user of health care with personal health needs or a partner in health care. As partners and participants in health care, carers may have little choice but to act as resources to fill in where health and social care provision is lacking. On the other hand, as clients or users of the service they have their own health needs and rights to a service. Indeed, they may wish to have their own health needs identified.

Meeting carers outside the home to discuss their own problems is one of the options that professionals should consider. At any time nurses should be prepared to take on the role of 'listening, clarifying and offering advice and information' as a provider of health care (Robinson and Yee 1991). Carers should be encouraged to identify their needs separately from those of the dependants, but this requires some sensitivity to the fact that carers may feel guilty and be reluctant to ask for help. Given that information about services has been identified as a major need of carers (Twigg 1992, Gunaratnum 1993), it is clearly another important aspect of the nurse's role to offer information in anticipation of carers' needs – something that has frequently been overlooked as an appropriate intervention (Badger *et al.* 1988).

Difficulties in working together

There are, however, some difficulties with this type of partnership. It may make more demands on families than they are willing to accept, or deny them the right to refuse. There is also an inherent tension between the professional and the carer in terms of equal status and power.

The ambiguity of the carer's position is decribed by Twigg in terms of the relationship between the professional and the carer (Twigg 1989). She describes ideal forms of relationships between carers and care-giving agencies: 'carers as resources', 'carers as co-workers' and 'carers as co-clients'. This classification emphasises and reinforces the different roles carers play, highlighting some of the contradictions in policy that see carers as a homogenous group. This frame of reference, described by Twigg, is applied to the findings in a study by Hearn (1993), who draws out the issues of participation in the relationships between district nurses and carers.

This small qualitative study is interesting and described in some detail as it draws out some important points about the ambiguity inherent in partnership. The study aims to explore the carers' perceptions of partnership with the district nurse. The findings show that, because district nurses were not able to control their workload, this had consequences for the increased involvement of the carer. Carers were acting as co-workers, not so much as a deliberate act of direction by the agency, but because the district nurse appeared to have little control over factors such as timing of visit or length of visit. This more common form of relationship between carer and nurse is described by the carer in terms of 'an apprentice' and 'the other nurse' (Hearn 1993). Rather than the relationship being based on equality it is based mainly on trust between carer and nurse. This trusting relationship allowed the carer to make decisions, such as how to lift the dependant, based upon own experience, rather than upon the professional knowledge communicated by the nurse. The carer often seemed to be carrying out tasks normally considered to be within the domain of the professional. Hearn (1993) further argued that carers had realistic expectations of the nurse and were aware of the seeming limitations the organisation put on the nurse, such as heavy caseloads and inability to make decisions about respite care. Carers perceived nurses as having little control over the services they were able to offer. In such situations carers tempered their own needs.

Thus the potential for participation in caring for the dependant is based on trust and enhanced by the shared lack of control that both nurse and carer have over the organisation. Hearn (1993) suggests that involvement which implies an active relationship might be a better word and a more realistic goal to strive for, rather than participation in care, which implies equal power and status that carers clearly do not have and may not want. As Hearn notes, 'participation with its inferences of power and equal status may be problematic in areas where control is not always preferred or possible' (Hearn 1993: 58).

It appears from this small family study that the carer gains from the role of co-worker if it is based on a relationship of trust that allows the carer to develop decision-making skills, to gain competence in caring tasks at an individual level and to enhance the feeling of control over the caring situation. Sharing professional knowledge with carers and recognising carers' own expertise are further ways in which involvement can be encouraged. Although the obligations carers feel towards their relatives need to be fulfilled, when the burden becomes too onerous it needs to be relieved. If nurses are not able to call on all the sources of care – state, private and voluntary – then they themselves will become unable to co-ordinate the care that is required. The danger of encouraging carers to become co-workers, however, is that then they might not be recognised as clients with their own health needs.

Support groups

Meeting carers' needs certainly involves talking to carers within the privacy of the home on an individual basis. Much may also be achieved through support groups, working on the principles of participation and involvement. Again, the provision may be inappropriate if dominated by professional perceptions of what is required. It seems that the best support groups are those that are based not only on what the group participants want, but also on the recognition of how groups develop and on the understanding of practical aspects of timing, location and transport.

An example of how involving carers as consumers in participation can founder is seen in the All Wales Strategy for Mentally Handicapped People. The carers in this case were parents and they were asked to participate in planning new services. Some of the characteristics of non-respondents are indicative of barriers to participation when setting up activities for carers

– the preoccupation with the day-to-day activities of caring leaving little time or energy for participation, well-established care routines with little desire for change, little knowledge of what the activity is about (McNaught 1991).

Establishing support groups is certainly a test of effectiveness, as carers may well vote with their feet and not attend. Patient satisfaction is a measurable outcome here. The ingredients of good support groups are documented by a small study of carers' groups carried out in one of the Inner London Boroughs (Morton and Mackenzie 1994). The study identified mutual support, social support, information resource, support from the group leader and the acknowledgement of carer status as the main positive aspects of support groups. A further interesting finding from this research was that the carer members of the group did not wish to take charge of the group themselves, but wanted to have someone else do the organising. They also felt that being supported and valued themselves was of importance. This sort of response echoes the fact that caring is an isolating activity, tiring and time consuming, leaving little energy for other demands. Coming to a group that someone else has organised is, for carers, a recognition of the contribution they are making to the health system.

The needs of group members also appeared to change over time. At the beginning of the group's life, members' primary needs were for information, friendship and social contact. The meeting was regarded as the social event in the week, 'something to look forward to', providing 'structure to the week' (Morton 1993: 64). In a longer-established group where the average membership was two years, members became more enthusiastic about lobbying for change and raising the profile of carers, compared to the group which had been formed only six months previously. Both groups studied catered for carers whose relatives had a range of health problems. This was seen as more advantageous and interesting than limiting groups to one diagnostic label such as stroke, since carers have many needs in common, the distinctions being based on kin relationships, culture and environment. All respondents in this study acknowledged the group leader's ability to work with them and sensitivity to their needs. The importance of not imposing professional ideas, such as promoting self-care, at a time when it is not appropriate was again demonstrated. Congruence in aims between group members and leaders is one key to success and incongruence is one of the reasons for failure.

An example of good practice that supports much of this research is noted by Chapman (1994), who describes the setting up of a support group for a locally identified need. In this group the district nurses acted as facilitators and resource agents. The group was set up with very limited financial resources and relied heavily upon the co-operation of voluntary agencies and the provision of cover for district nurses' time spent on the project. Evaluations of such ventures demonstrate the need for support groups to be given appropriate resources and to be incorporated into service provision, if they are to be of lasting value to carers.

Conclusion

It seems that caring may become dysfunctional and be as chronic a condition for the carer as the disability is for the dependent relative or receiver of care. Evidence from support groups and from carers' graphic descriptions of the imposed changes in life-style and of the never-ending task of caring, together with the emotional stress of changed relationships, echoes the uncertain and long-term goals of chronic illness. The interplay between task and feelings may sustain, as well as be stressful to, both carer and dependant. This complex relationship must be recognised by primary health care nurses.

Assessing needs of carers should take into account not only the tasks and burdens of caring, but also the kinship ties and cultural environments in which the care takes place. We have to recognise that handicap is culturally and socially defined. Simply concluding from the evidence in a wealth of literature that carers find the burden of caring difficult is likely to lead to a labelling of carers in the same way that 'the disabled' are labelled. It is quite feasible that some carers may manage very well with small but regular respite care, or with the service of someone who can compensate for routine and daily acts of living such as dressing (Oliver 1988).

While the surveys of consumers that describe types of carer, identify gaps in service and draw conclusions about service provision are very useful, so too are the smaller-scale studies which draw out from carers' own experiences the details of their day-to-day life. Further work also needs to be done on the practice areas of nursing in order to show how effective such practices are. Clearly some resources are more useful than others. For instance, much might be learned from the All Wales Strategy for Mentally Handicapped People about what sort of service is likely to work. Also, further evaluations of the practices of support groups or of initiatives that are taken by nurses will help to make more appropriate assessments and to incorporate some assessments into everyday practice. Case-finding activities will also help to identify those who are not in contact with community services through the usual referral systems.

The large surveys have noted the similarities among carers and also highlighted the differences. It also seems, however, that there are common needs both within population groups and across groups such as white, black and Chinese populations. All have a need for appropriate information, acceptable respite and accessible services. Such common needs are a starting point for providers and for purchasers, but the satisfaction for carers will be determined by how far these needs are properly interpreted and provided for within the context of the culture and of individual families. Incorporating the needs of carers into service provision has yet to be achieved (Twigg 1993). Caring means a relationship and infers dependency to a greater or lesser degree. Caring should only be assessed as part of that relationship. It must always be seen in its context and the effectiveness of services must likewise be measured.

The ambiguous position of carers as both providers of care and as clients makes them vulnerable to abuse by purchasers, who may see them as a cheap option and not recognise their needs as clients. Accepting help is also not easy for carers who feel an obligation towards their relatives or friends and genuinely want to care for them. Both situations have to be provided for and realistic choices should be available. If a service is unacceptable, then carers have no choice.

Nurses working in this context are in an advantageous position to take on the assessment and evaluation of provision in primary health care. They may not be the main providers, but they have entry into the private domain of the home where care is carried out, and are therefore in key positions to assess the burden and the relief needed and not only to provide a service, but also to identify need for purchasers and commissioners.

Chapter 7
New nursing roles in primary health care

Summary

This chapter addresses the challenge of developing new roles for primary health care nurses within the context of purchasing, providing and contracting. The professional initiatives and policies that are enabling and influencing changes in role are examined, together with the tensions arising from the conflict between individual and community approaches. The effects of the changing role on practice are discussed, with particular reference to increasing autonomy through nursing development units and redefinition of roles, seen in moves towards nurse prescribing, development of nurse practitioners and the increase of practice nurses.

Purchasing and providing

The development of new nursing roles is made legitimate by a policy that demands increased accessibility to health care, improved quality, closer interprofessional working and cost-effective professional skill mix. Increasingly primary care is becoming a focal point of health care provision. The expansion of the GP fundholding scheme and primary care-led purchasing (Carruthers 1994) means that nurses have great opportunities for developing practice. Joining together of District Health Authorities (DHAs) and Family Health Services Authorities (FHSAs) into local commissioning health authorities means that GPs and fundholding practices will be able to extend their role in contracting. Decentralisation of decision making and the different approaches to health care delivery by organisations such as Trusts, GP fundholders and the independent sector will further facilitate a diversity of nursing roles.

Carruthers (1994) gives examples of how primary care-led purchasing may be achieved. He emphasises the importance of clarifying the roles of fundholders, non-fundholding practices and local commissioning Health Authorities, and the use of both quantitative and qualitative information of clinically effective practice to develop contract specifications. Understanding and responding to the different needs and expectations of the user entails making the best use of people through the development of skills and teamwork. Further government initiatives, such as the setting of targets in *Health of the Nation* (DoH 1992), give impetus for health-promoting activities and healthy alliances. It seems, however, that purchasers have differing views of how nurses should be involved in contracting. In a study of the implications of contracting for district nurses, Smith *et al.* (1993) discovered that there was ambivalence on the part of purchasers about the extent to which nurses should be involved. Some valued the district nurses' knowledge about the community and saw them as able not only to identify needs, but also to make suggestions about provision. Others saw the nurses' viewpoint as biased and protective of their own professionalism. The result of these different perspectives may be, on the one hand, a tight prescriptive task-related contract or, on the other, a contract that reflects the nurses' perspectives of needs and includes evaluation of new practices. The latter will challenge nurses to be involved beyond provision of care.

In this way nurses working with practice populations and local communities have the chance to influence the contracting process. Their position of being close to the local population means that they are able not only to communicate the needs of patients, but also to suggest ways in which services might be provided and to prove the worth of these suggestions in practice. Epidemiological data about the population will be drawn from a number of sources, as discussed in Chapter 2, but not least from the primary health care nurse's 'intimate knowledge of the neighbourhood' (Gillam *et al.* 1994:12), recorded in practice profiles and documented in caseload and workload profiles. Clearly, service specifications need to take account of data collected by nurses. Together these quantitative and qualitative sources provide the basis for identifying needs, evaluating provision and changing the ways in which care is delivered.

Nurses themselves are demonstrating the importance of new roles through practice (Ross and Elliott 1995). District nurses are taking on the challenges of community-based assessments and acknowledging the importance of taking health promotion initiatives rather than making referrals to others. Health visitors are redefining their role and re-establishing their practice in public health. Community psychiatric nurses are moving their focus of practice from hospital to primary health.

The Tile Hill project in Coventry (Reid 1993) provides an example of district nurses, health visitors, community psychiatric nurses and other grades of staff working together with GPs, using the GP-managed primary health care team model from the Roy Report (1990) as inspiration. The unit offers all nursing staff the chance to develop their own specialism and to be part of a team acting as a nursing provider unit working with local GPs. One of the reported strengths of this unit is the skill mix that has been determined by the nurses themselves rather than imposed by management. Another initiative has been the development of patient-held notes that are multi-disciplinary. The contracting process demands value for money and a cost-effective service, and is a stimulus for addressing skill mix.

Skill mix

The issue of skill mix in primary health care nursing is part of the wider interest in skill mix of all professional roles in health care. This is nothing new. Over 20 years ago Hockey (1972) was arguing that district nurses were overtrained for part of their role.

The skill mix review by the NHS Management Executive (NHSME 1992) achieved notoriety for its concentration on grade mix and cost cutting, rather than on quality and health gain. The responses from professional organisations demonstrated that skill mix and grade review are contentious issues if the only rationale is to save money (Mackenzie and Cowley 1993). In the context of contracting, however, it is important to recognise the appropriate use of staff. Substitution of skills, that is, 'matching skills to work within and across professions' (NAHAT 1993: 13), has to be based on population needs and seen as the opportunity to indulge in new practice. Both substitution and development of role may result in skill mix review (Gibbs *et al.* 1991).

One of the dangers of skill mix is that it will be used to cut costs by reducing staff numbers, particularly the higher more expensive grades. It therefore becomes entangled in grading issues rather than in matching skills to health needs. Top-down approaches by management are not as acceptable as that illustrated by the Tile Hill project, whereby priorities, activities and responsibilities are reviewed by the multi-disciplinary team itself. This approach takes into account that nurses work in an interprofessional team and not in isolation. Indeed skill mix reviews in primary health care teams should include not only nurses, but also GPs, administrative staff and health care assistants.

Developing new roles will require greater understanding and more openness on the part of nurses to try out new ways, rather than working to prescribed job descriptions. An increased confidence will be required to negotiate roles that do not rely on delegated tasks as previously (Bowling 1985). Negotiation will result in clinical protocols outlining boundaries of responsibility. The danger is that protocols may just become another version of delegated task-driven duties, if nurses are not able to state with confidence the extent of their contribution to health in terms of health gains. In relation to practice, some examples of protocols or clinical guidelines are now being published nationally and have the benefit of the experience and expertise of multidisciplinary working groups. One example is that of cancer pain management, including audit (Working Party on Clinical Guidelines in Palliative Care 1994), which describes how doctors, district nurses, specialist nurses, spiritual advisers, social workers and voluntary workers might co-operate with each other and the patient and family to manage pain.

Skill mix is also a response to the *Strategy for Nursing's* (DoH 1989a) call for the agreement of numbers and deployment of staff in all health care settings (Target 17). The introduction of Project 2000 will enable nurses to work, at an RGN level, in primary health care teams. They will become as important a nursing resource as practice nurses working within the general practice team. Decentralisation of services has also offered the impetus to make good use of resources. A review of skills will be done effectively only if health gain for the population is the goal and if nurses themselves are involved. Such an approach was used in Islington where information was used to make decisions about staff allocation and resourcing (Drennan 1990a, b). Determining skill mix in terms of quality of care and patient outcomes, however, is difficult to establish. This accounts for the fact that most of the skill mix reviews have concentrated on tasks.

Increasing autonomy in professional practice

Additional to the changes in health policy and legislation are changes in the nursing profession that seem set to acknowledge the new roles for nurses and enhance autonomy. *The Scope of Professional Practice* (UKCC 1992) gives nurses confidence to challenge the traditional restrictions on extended clinical roles, which were previously defined by the DHSS (1977) and sometimes implemented through inflexible management. As a result of increasing autonomy, changes in community management and interprofessional team working, there will be greater demands on experienced and qualified nurses in the community to act in a supervisory capacity, not only for others in the nursing team, but also for other professional colleagues. The importance of clinical supervision, defined by Faugier (1994: 64) as 'the activity of examining one's practice with a more experienced and skilled professional in a formal relationship', was noted by the review of mental health nursing (DoH 1994b). The main purpose of clinical supervision is to improve the quality of patient care by the educative process of developing skills, by the support of colleagues and other professionals and by the monitoring and improvement of staff performance (Kohner 1994).

Clinical supervision raises issues of resources in terms of time and skills, if the functions are to be carried out appropriately. As Faugier (1994) notes, clinical supervision requires sensitivity and skill over and above that required for patient or client interactions, otherwise it will not be effective in facilitating reflective practice and in offering guidance. There is a danger too that the word supervision will be interpreted by nurses as staff appraisal or individual performance review. Although there may be links, definitions and purposes need to be made clear in order to distinguish the activities.

The Stepney Neighbourhood Nursing Team (Kohner 1994) has used other terminology in order to clarify this distinction, preferring the term active management to clinical supervision. In this example the manager is the clinical supervisor and this perhaps accounts for the different terminology. In such situations it is highly likely that there will be confusion, and managers may be better advised to develop the supervisory capacity of their clinical staff, rather than to take on the role themselves. Clinical supervision is also used in education, where the supervisor is a teacher in the clinical setting. This is a familiar situation in district nursing, health visiting and community psychiatric nursing. Whether or not clinical supervision focuses on developing new areas of practice, or on monitoring and improving staff performance, it is part of assuring quality and is consequent on continuing education (UKCC 1995).

Changes in the educational preparation for community health care nursing (UKCC 1991, 1994) also open the way for existing community nurses, such as district nurses, health visitors, community psychiatric nurses, school nurses and occupational health nurses, to explore new roles in their areas of specialism and expertise. It is important and timely that practice nurses are now established within the specialisation of community health care nursing (UKCC 1994). This specialisation is recognition of the additional education following registration required by nurses who wish to practise as specialist nursing practitioners (UKCC 1994). In the community this level of practice will be required for a range of discrete areas of specialist nursing practice, described by the UKCC (1994) as general practice nursing, community mental health nursing, community mental handicap nursing, community children's nursing, public health nursing – health visiting, occupational health nursing, nursing in the home – district nursing and school nursing. These rather unwieldy titles incorporate the current areas of practice as well as new titles to be included on the register, reflecting the concern of practising nurses that their specific contributions to community nursing will be lost in this all-encompassing term of community health care nursing.

The proposals for community education (UKCC 1991) are part of the Council's project on post-registration education and practice (PREPP) and call for a new type of education based on 'core skills with additional discrete modules necessary for functioning in specific roles to meet specific needs' (UKCC 1991: 9). The proposals acknowledge the complexity of community care and describe a range of activities, from simple assistance with physical activities to complex psychological, social and emergency interventions. The proposals recognise that community health care nursing is concerned with the social and health needs of individuals, groups and communities, based on the following principles:

- practitioners who are prepared to be accountable and respect the vulnerability and primacy of those requiring health care
- quality service
- support of carers
- reducing inequality in access and care provision

- effective multi-disciplinary and multi-agency co-operation
- cost effectiveness of policies and services

(UKCC 1991: para.13: 11)

These principles represent a welcome change as a starting point for curricula and are not intended to be prescriptive. They may lead to a number of curriculum models to meet local needs, but still maintain some measure of comparability across courses. Although the proposals may be criticised for lacking clarity in terminology, for rationalising roles and education in community nursing and for moving towards general isolation and fragmentation, with clinical specialists being developed to fill the gaps, nevertheless the opportunities presented far outweigh the concerns. The proposals offer a broader vision of health care professionals working together to meet social and health care needs and will encourage more flexible practice, the potential for a single point of user contact with nurses in the primary health care team and a challenge to tribalism.

The subsequent report (UKCC 1994), outlining the learning outcomes for curricula, does not fully achieve the hoped-for flexibility promised in the initial proposals, but tends to identify boundaries between the specialist groups. None the less it is a promising start for educators and practitioners. Educators will also need to consider how experience in practice settings contributes to learning, given research findings that demonstrate the importance of well-qualified clinical supervisors, together with an environment that fosters learning and risk taking, in enabling community health care nurses to work in the uncertainty of primary health (Mackenzie 1992, Twinn 1989). It is in the real world of practice situations that continuing education is able to achieve the hoped-for analytical, thinking and knowledgeable practitioner, who is able to deal with the uncertain and 'messy' problems of practice (Schon 1987).

The influences of contracting, however, are as great in education as anywhere else in the health service. Higher education too is part of the market place and has to entice commissioners to support student numbers. Educators' best intentions may well be to meet educational aims, but they must take notice of purchasers who want courses to meet the service demands. In order to ensure a properly qualifed workforce, contracts must include a statement about the adequacy of education for all levels of practice, otherwise costs will dictate the provision of education and consequently reduce the quality of practice. Such contracts would overcome the lack of ring-fenced money for continuing education and oblige Trusts and GP fundholders to pay for courses that prepare nurses properly for practice in primary health. Educators for their part need to be innovative in their curriculum planning and offer flexible courses that meet a variety of needs without compromising standards. Fears of territorialism will have to be set aside and the best of interprofessional education accepted. Educators themselves need to re-think their approaches to practice and embrace new ways of working and thinking.

The difficulties of tribalism and of adherence to traditional practices among nurses, their teachers and managers have been barriers to innovation and change, causing Cumberlege (1986) to suggest that practitioners should practise their skills based on the assessed needs of the community and neighbourhood and should work alongside general practitioners. Contracts will state not only what is to be provided but also the level of education and preparation needed to be able to carry out a particular role. For instance, if nurses are to visit at home they must have the necessary educational preparation to assess the family and work unsupervised. Given all that has been said before, this may sound like professional protection, but it is fundamental to giving a quality service and protecting the patient or client. In this instance nurses have to take on the issues of responsibility and accountability and nowhere is this more obvious than in nurse prescribing.

Nurse prescribing

In itself nurse prescribing is not a radical departure from current practice, because at present the prescribable products are mostly over-the-counter medicines and because it only legitimises the decision making and professional judgement already taking place. It would be a mistake, however, if nurses were to use prescribing as a status symbol enhancing nursing power and status in relation to medicine. It should be seen as increasing the range of services and accessibility of treatment for the patient.

If nurses are to exploit their new role in nurse prescribing for the benefit of the patient, and also ensure safety, it is essential that there is good communication between the nurse, the GP, the pharmacist and, where appropriate, other agencies such as hospitals, hospices and day hospitals. Nurses in primary care, pharmacists and GPs share many patients. Their different contributions to health care should be monitored through the judicious use of protocols. This raises questions about information sharing, records and referral mechanisms. It is widely accepted that all areas have shortcomings. Ross (1989) found that GPs and district nurses looking after the same patients, and in principle having access to shared medical and nursing records, were in the majority of cases at some disagreement about the prescribed medication. It is in the assessment that information sharing between professionals is crucial. Knowledge of the patients' previous and current medication for present and previous conditions, as well as of drug sensitivities and allergies, is essential to all carers at the outset. Clinical decisions also have to be made about whether or not drug therapy is the most appropriate option. This new legislation is a recognition and legitimation of the nurse's prescribing role, and demonstrates confidence in practice accountability. Nurses must ensure that they have the necessary comprehensive education to carry out the new role and must learn from the pilot sites involved in the implementation.

An example of nurse prescribing is described by Emmerson (1994) in respect of delivering health care to homeless people. This project recognises the importance of communicating with a wide range of professionals, including pharmacists from the Trust and the FHSA. Protocols are established, following careful planning and discussion, and are used in a positive way to guide practice and set it within legislation. Practitioners undertake an education course that prepares them for autonomous decision making and protects the client from unsafe practice.

Nursing development units

The King's Fund and through it the Department of Health have encouraged the movement of nurse autonomy through their support and funding of Nurse Development Units (NDU) (Vaughan 1994). Since the first NDU was established in the early 1980s by Alan Pearson they had increased to about 300 in Great Britain by 1992, although there are still few examples in primary health care. One notable exception comes from Northern Ireland where nurses have set up four research-based projects:

- assessment of the need for a carers' support group
- evaluation of the role of the diabetic liaison nurse
- evaluation of ongoing therapy sessions with patients with chronic mental illness
- a holistically based assessment of the needs of pregnant teenagers

(Mason and Beattie 1993)

In a funded NDU project in Nottingham the issues health visitors are attempting to address include poor mental health in women, increased violence against women, provision for young children under 8 years, improving liaison with the housing department and solvent abuse training for health workers. These issues are based on data collected from the local population and are a response to local need. In this project health visitors are not only giving support and advice but also facilitating other community workers and clients to set up projects (Boyd *et al.* 1993).

Such units demonstrate the special contributions that nurses are able to make to assessing and promoting health and to evaluating their value to health care. A further development is the redefinition of role encompassed in the movement towards nurse practitioner.

Redefinition of role – the nurse practitioner

The nurse practitioner has been described as one way in which nurses in primary health care might redefine their role (Trnobranski 1994).

The term nurse practitioner embraces a number of aspects such as:

- assessment including physical examination and history taking
- management of illness and continuity of care
- health promotion and support
- collaboration with physicians and other health workers to provide co-ordinated care
- provision of specialist services for defined groups

One of the characteristics differentiating nurse practitioners in primary health care teams from other nurses, according to Stilwell (1992), is that they are the first point of contact for the patient and hence are dealing with undifferentiated health problems for which they need to make a nursing diagnosis. They work within the team according to protocols and therefore it seems they are equal members.

The associated innovations in practice are seen as a necessary response to demographic and epidemiological changes and to technological advance (WHO 1989). The nurse practitioner role might be seen as affording opportunities to develop the nurse's role, thus giving a choice to patients and a more accessible, acceptable service – pioneered in the community setting by Burke Masters (1987), Stilwell *et al.* (1987) and Atkinson (1987). Less positively, nurse practitioners might be seen as substituting inadequately for the doctor.

Bryar (1994) describes the following influences on the nurse practitioner role:

- demands to meet the needs of disadvantaged groups in the community such as homeless people
- demands to contain health care costs

- increasing maturity and confidence of community nurses in developing new roles
- emphasis at the international level on a model of community-based PHC that makes explicit the nurse's role in PHC

To these might be added:

- inappropriate use of medical and nursing manpower and skills
- expectations for improved services such as shorter waiting times
- strong influence from professional nursing groups
- quality of care initiatives
- need for increased accessibility

Redefining the role in this way may also result in another round of new terminology and re-establishment of boundaries. For instance, Bryar (1994) calls for a differentiation of roles between public health nurses and nurse practitioners. According to Bryar, the public health role involves identifying and monitoring health needs, whereas the nurse practitioner provides services that meet needs identified by individuals. This concern for differentiation of role is likely to lead to another bout of tribalism and concern for new labels based on what nurses do rather than on what patients and clients need. On a more helpful note, Bryar (1994) also suggests that primary health care nurses are likely to be fulfilling much of the role of a nurse practitioner, or at least have the potential to do so, and that before any new nurses are employed the resources of present nurses and their skills should be assessed together with their potential. The recent Touche Ross (1994) evaluation supports this.

There are numerous instances of nurses working in what might be regarded as an expanded role in response to local needs, and so meeting the characteristics of a nurse practitioner described above. The Hospital at Home Scheme, started in the 1980s in

Peterborough, was one such scheme that has been used as a model for others. Hospital at Home (Mackenzie 1991) was incorporated into the mainstream of provision following initial pilot work, demonstrating how, with facilitative management and appropriate skill mix, patients can be discharged from hospital early into the care of district nurses working in close contact with the hospital and the GP.

Many would agree that district nurses, health visitors, community psychiatric nurses and a range of other nurses practising independently, autonomously and seeing patients with undifferentiated health problems in primary health could be called nurse practitioners. Indeed the UKCC (1991) has argued for abolishing the term nurse practitioner and resisting yet another title in nursing. It is unlikely, however, that nursing will be able to accept that, obsessed as it is with titles to defend and define practice within the profession.

Professionalisation issues such as this, however, are not likely to be a major justification for this role in the face of cost effectiveness, unless they can be linked with the arguments of quality and health gain. The importance of research to demonstrate outcome will be the most convincing way of furthering the role of the nurse practitioner and has been an important issue in the USA (Molde and Diers 1985, Stone 1994).

A review of the American and British literature indicates that during the 1970s and early 1980s there was considerable debate and research into the role of the nurse practitioner in the USA. These studies focused on:

- acceptability to patient/physicians
- the work environment
- health outcomes
- cost
- effect of educational background
- style of practice

One of the best-known studies is sometimes known as the Burlington randomised controlled trial (Spitzer *et al.* 1974). This early evaluation study consisted of the random allocation of patients to a nurse practitioner or a doctor for any first contact. In a total of 392 episodes of care the nurse management was rated as adequate in 69 per cent of cases compared with 66 per cent in the doctor group. Nurse practitioners were able to function independently in 67 per cent of the patient contacts, and the vast majority of patients (96 per cent) were satisfied with seeing the nurse. Subsequent studies in the USA, and the most comprehensive so far, have found some evidence to show that nurse practitioners are acceptable to patients and physicians, improve accessibility of health care services, improve productivity of practice and medical services and therefore reduce costs (Congress of the United States 1986).

In Britain, evaluation studies have focused on small-scale or single nurse practitioner innovations. The study in Birmingham is the best known (Stilwell 1984). This study suggests that the focus of the nurse practitioner's work in general practice is holistic care of the client. The assessment and treatment is broader based than the doctor's, and includes concerns with rehabilitation, coping and the psycho-social aspects of illness. More recently, South East Thames Regional Health Authority (SETRHA 1993) secured funding for evaluating 20 nurse practitioners, the aim being to test the hypothesis that a major part of health care needs in primary health can be met effectively and efficiently by nurse practitioners.

The evaluation of these pilot projects (Touche Ross 1994) particularly addressed patient satisfaction, resource effectiveness and practitioner performance. They did not, however, look at cost effectiveness, in the absence of agreed outcome measures. This is an important study as it is the first major UK study of nurse practitioners in a diversity of sites: open access community settings, accident and emergency departments, primary care alongside GPs. The latter, the report concludes, 'is where there is greatest scope for the development of the nurse practitioner in managing a comprehensive caseload jointly with GPs . . . this needs to be taken forward within a wider debate on the objectives, staffing and skill mix for primary care' (Touche Ross 1994). Nurse practitioners achieved high levels of patient satisfaction in all sites. In the community sites they were most valuable in filling the care gap for unregistered patients in a homeless care project, thus reinforcing the value of previous work (Burke Masters 1987, Atkinson 1987). In other community sites, such as the retail chemist, the full range of nurse practitioner skills were less likely to be used at this stage and were therefore of less value in filling the care gap. Accident and emergency sites offered a clearly defined role in the management of minor injuries, rather than severe illness and injury. Here and in the primary care sites the nurse practitioners were found to provide a safe, valued and beneficial service to selected groups of patients. In the community sites it was concluded that an enhanced district nurse and health visitor role could more usefully provide the services needed and support other initiatives (Atkinson 1987, Baker 1994). Further research will be necessary to evaluate the work of qualified and experienced nurse practitioners as these posts become established. As the report (Touche Ross 1994) notes, the most experienced practitioners were able to practise in a way that reduced some elements of the cost of care and this needs to be investigated.

Clearly, Health Authorities regard the measurement of nurse practitioner interventions as imperative, but evaluation is not without difficulties and presents methodological issues for researchers, particularly when addressing quality. Suitable indicators of quality that measure the results of nursing interventions on patient outcomes are difficult to isolate when the nurse is working as a member of an interprofessional team. The introduction of protocols that identify the parameters of care and concentrate on process criteria will not give an accurate indication of nurse practitioners' effectiveness in terms of patient outcomes, that is benefit to the patient or client, but are more likely to measure compliance with the protocol. Other difficulties that will need to be addressed will be the differences between the doctors' work and the nurses' before comparative studies can be set up, as they will be unlikely to compare like with like. Indeed, there will be differences among the caseloads of nurse practitioners. For instance, some may be dealing with long-term health problems, some with acute care such as early discharge following surgery, and other caseloads may include paediatric care where parents may be as much the user of the service as is the child. Social circumstances, ethnic and cultural background will be variables of equal importance to diagnosis, age and surgical operation. In this respect the criteria for patient satisfaction may not be transferable across cultures as a measure of accessibility or acceptability, as some cultures do not value seeing the nurse in preference to the doctor. Community nurses will need to be involved in isolating outcome criteria to measure effectiveness and efficiency, in addition to those in general use, i.e. readmission rates or waiting times.

Specialist nurses

The expansion of nurse practitioners into both specialist and generalist areas is to be welcomed and hopefully will dispel some of the differences about the value of specialists and generalists in community nursing. The ten government-funded nurse practitioner posts announced in 1994 (Day 1994) cover a wide range of practice in different settings, involving specialist areas such as patients with glaucoma and rheumatism to a more general role working as part of a team in an inner-city health centre.

The comparisons between nurse specialist and nurse generalist have been much debated in the USA (Holt 1987) reflecting similar problems to those in the UK. It is interesting to note that the nurse practitioner has lagged behind the clinical nurse specialist in the USA, due to the close alignment with the physician for education and practice. Clinical nurse specialists, on the other hand, have made nursing practice their area of independence from the start and have been educated through masters programmes. While both roles are now merging, there are some lessons to be learned in the UK from their development: firstly, that education is important to underpin practice; secondly, that autonomy within the role is essential for the development of practice; and finally that interprofessional working is more important than individual practice in health care today. To this end nurse practitioners in the UK must be confident without being defensive about their roles in relation to doctors and others in their own profession.

In an effort to outline the expanding activities for primary health care teams, NAHAT (1993) describes them in terms of medical specialities, such as genito-urinary medicine or gynaecology. The enthusiasm for expansion of health care into the community could mean that nurses' roles are determined by clinical specialisation and medical diagnosis rather than by the need to consider new ways of meeting the health needs of a population. The development of nurse practitioners, or nurses using that term, however, spans both generalist and specialist roles, as previously noted. One does not need to exclude the other.

An example of the specialisation in the generalist field of district nursing and health visiting comes from Scotland (Baker 1994). In response to the health needs of people with HIV infection and AIDS, a district nurse and a health visitor have developed their skills in the specialist area of HIV. As a result there has been improved liaison and co-ordination between hospital and other agencies and provision of education to community staff, with consequent improvement of services to the patients and clients. Funded research is also linked to this project, which will help evaluation. Both specialist and generalist roles have a place in needs-led practice.

From the experiences in the USA education clearly has a role in determining the level of autonomy and independence that nurses can achieve. In this respect the practice nurse would seem to be the most vulnerable to medical domination and task-orientated practice in the UK.

Practice nurses

The increasing numbers of practice nurses (Stilwell 1991), together with concerns about their educational preparation, add to the drive for a new practitioner who will work more closely with the GP than district nurses and health visitors have done previously. In a National Census in 1990 it was reported there were 7,520 practice nurses, representing 20 per cent of nurses, working in the primary health care team (Atkin and Lunt 1993).

Changes in the GP Contract introduced in 1990 have encouraged practice nurses to look for a more autonomous and different role in the practice team. This is mainly in response to the increasing demands for screening and primary prevention being largely delegated to practice nurses. In this situation the term nurse practitioner is appealing and to some extent has furthered the cause of nurse practitioners. The role of practice nurses is not well focused, however, and the activities they engage in are wide ranging. In a study by Ross *et al.* (1994) the tasks of 620 practice nurses in one health region ranged from primary prevention, of which 92.9 per cent gave travel immunisations and 76 per cent gave child immunisations, to administrative tasks such as stocktaking and cleaning. Nurses were often the first point of contact with the public, giving telephone advice on clinical matters, dealing with emergencies and giving first aid. In addition, 66.9 per cent of nurses also set up health promotion clinics and were responsible for the call/recall system. Some also supported the GP and acted as chaperones. The majority wanted to develop their participation in health promotion and counselling, which they regarded as important to their role. As only 6 per cent of the respondents had a health visiting qualification and 13 per cent a district nursing qualification, a large number of practice nurses in this region were not well prepared for the broad range of tasks they were undertaking. On the other hand, all were overqualified for tasks such as cleaning and chaperoning.

The diversity of activity is also noted by Bradford and Winn (1993). In a study of 65 practice nurses in Brighton it was clear that the majority would like more education on health promotion or clinical aspects and counselling. The health promotion activities were largely carried out in the form of health promotion clinics, such as clinics for diabetes or asthma, from which it is concluded that this work is more about disease management than primary prevention. The practice nurses' views about health promotion are not exclusively concerned with just changing behaviour or medical intervention, but the research also indicates that practice nurses are in agreement with more radical models that enable patients and clients to make informed choices and involve influencing health promotion through political and social environments.

A further study (Ochera *et al.* 1993) shows that health promotion work in the form of health checks is carried out exclusively by practice nurses. While this study concludes that the future expansion of role for practice nurses could be in health promotion, research also demonstrates the diversity of activity in this role, which reflects the vagaries of policy and GP contracts. In such a situation the practice nurses' role may expand and contract in response to policy, rather than be led by the nurses' own recognition of their contribution to the community's health, despite the potential and the recognition of the limitation of the activities in which they are engaged (Ochera *et al.* 1993). This study recommends more emphasis on outcome studies of the effectiveness of practice nurses, adding to the small amount of work already started (British Heart Family Study 1994).

Practice nurses will also have a major role to play in general practice audit, co-operating with GPs and other health professionals. Audit in general practice is well established but is only recently extending to include interprofessional audit. Examples of audit are now available drawing on the specialist experience of advisory groups. One such involves practice nurses, GPs and others working together in the management of diabetes (British Diabetic Association 1993).

Tensions between individual and community approaches

One of the tensions in nursing in primary health care that has made changes in practice difficult to implement has been between the individualised and the community approach. Nursing itself concentrates on a holistic, individualised approach to care, identifying individual health problems, which not only assumes that there is a clear-cut answer to the problems, but also implies that ill health is the concern of individual action. In an effort to analyse policy and practice, Beattie (1991) has conceptualised alternative approaches to this concentration on top–down action that concentrates on persuading people to modify their behaviour and change their life-style. He suggests a number of other approaches to promoting health that involve professionals in a negotiated relationship – 'a personal counselling for health' model or a 'community development' for health approach. Both involve individuals taking their own action rather than being in the position of having to change their life-style, without help or in situations that are not easy to change. For instance, reducing smoking or alcohol intake is not easy without help and support (Beattie 1991). In such situations, nurses will need to change their role in relation to the patient or client as well as to other professionals. This change in role is not just applicable to primary or secondary prevention, but also to the maintenence of care with those who have a disability and handicap. The changes in role are concerned with altering not just the ways of working or the tasks, but also the approach to health.

It is not that there has to be a distinction between the individual approach and the community approach or group approach, but rather a difference in the relationship between the patient or client and the practitioner. Here lies the nub of the change – a different way of thinking about how health can be achieved and maintained and how the nurse can contribute. Working with individuals is important, but it is not enough. There also has to be a recognition by nurses that they can take personal responsibility for initiating interventions, rather than waiting to be told what to do. The emphasis in general practice on responding to individuals has also influenced nursing. Therefore the practice team as a whole will need a more rigorous approach towards developing needs assessment and will need to 'combine the best of demand-led personal care with the population focus required to develop a needs-led service' (Plamping 1994).

Conclusion

The contract culture has coincided with the profession's moves towards autonomous roles and, as practice examples show, the opportunities presented have been seized by nurses in primary care. New roles in practice will inevitably involve change, some of which will be traumatic, but much will be motivating, and for those who can grasp the chance it will be a positive experience. Many of the innovations described in the literature are small scale and unevaluated. If they are to be of lasting value and of interest to purchasers, they must be incorporated into the mainstream of provision and their effectiveness evaluated, otherwise some very good ideas will be lost.

Among all this enthusiasm the dangers of contracting, which may lead to cost effectiveness without paying heed to quality, need to be recognised. Primary health care nurses are in positions to influence contracts and to ensure, for instance, that statements about education are included as a means to protect standards and patients.

The shift in power from Health Authorities to GP fund-holders is a positive aspect of the reforms. The energies expended by nurses in the past in trying to work between the demands of management and GPs can now be used to specify their contribution to the team and to negotiate their role on the basis of population needs. Interprofessional activities in clinical audit will be part of a review that encompasses all members of the primary health care team including GPs, administrative staff and health care assistants, and uses patient and client outcomes as a measure, so necessary in the present climate. Hopefully this will lead to greater autonomy, improved morale and interprofessional co-operation.

Chapter 8
Conclusion and future directions

This conclusion aims to draw together the themes in this book and to summarise the major implications for present and future nursing practice in primary health care.

Throughout this book we have highlighted the positive role primary health care nurses can play. They are in a position to make a major contribution to the overall audit of community health needs and, by working closely with other professionals and family carers, to make a comprehensive assessment of individual needs and to ensure the best use of resources in order to deliver the highest possible quality of care. In fact, we have argued, they can be the initiators of change, the pioneers of quality, and lead primary care towards a user-centred and fully integrated service.

In order to achieve this it is necessary to work with patients, clients or users in imaginative ways, combining experience and expertise with other health care professionals and agencies. Such initiatives cannot, however, be carried out in isolation or without regard to policy, which pervades and influences all of health care in the UK. A greater understanding of policy should therefore help primary health nurses to exert their own influence and to work towards a more responsive and less rigid system.

Assessment is the starting point for many health activities and initiates provision. It may be regarded as the precursor for all health care planning at a population and individual level, as discussed in the two complementary chapters on health-needs profiling and assessment, although, as we have noted, health-needs assessment is an inexact science. Such shortcomings need to be recognised by nurses in primary health care who are trying to combine and compare local and national health data and to use it to consider priorities. The use of health profiles of populations, however, may well be a better guide to the needs of the community and a better guide to meeting health needs than the vagaries of policy directives.

Recent legislation has made the GP the linchpin in the reforms in primary health care, having fundholding responsibilities and fulfilling both a puchaser and provider role. Nurses in primary health care should not be daunted by this change, but should recognise the opportunities it offers them to influence the service. Alongside this role come strong guidelines for improving the responsiveness of services to consumer needs, allowing the consumer choice and increasing value for money and standards of care. The resulting contracts offer a real opportunity for nurses to build in some control in relation to ensuring quality that has to do with user satisfaction, needs of carers and needs of groups outside the mainstream of provision.

Benefits for patients will be greater if nurses exercising this control have received a level of education and training commensurate with their new responsibilities. In this respect, it is important that continuing nurse education funding is not competing with the demands of service and that the requisite level of education for nurses in primary health care is stated in contracts. Working within general practice at a level of interprofessional co-operation will initiate joint projects of innovation and evaluation and subsequently achieve the better collaboration and interprofessional co-operation that primary health care requires.

Nursing is often a hidden activity and needs to be made more visible to purchasers and commissioners through the specifications drawn up by providers. One way forward is to evaluate the innovations now being carried out in primary health care nursing. In the review of innovations carried out for this book (Ross and Elliott 1995) it is noteworthy that very few of the projects are designed to be outcome based or evaluated. There remain many issues to be resolved and much research yet to do particularly in the areas of teamwork effectiveness and patient outcomes.

The importance of measuring outcomes cannot be ignored, as has been noted in discussing quality assurance, interprofessional audits and the development of new roles. There has, however, been very little practice evaluation and research on outcomes in primary health care nursing. There are a number of reasons for this. Firstly, the outcomes and baseline need defining. This is sometimes difficult when health problems are multi-faceted and complex and do not always have clear-cut solutions, particularly in situations of continuing care needs. Secondly, there is an increasing trend towards the use of qualitative research methods in nursing, which also limits outcome-based research, because of the small numbers involved and the inappropriateness of generalisation. Neither of these are excuses for not engaging in outcome measurement. Indeed, in-depth research studies may well be the most appropriate first step and could be used to identify suitable indicators for patient outcomes or be part of a larger evaluation study.

Outcomes and cost measurement are in direct contrast to the caring that many nurses regard as a central part of giving quality care. They are not, however, incompatible.

Any book that is written from a policy perspective gets quickly out of date. Inevitably there will be shifts in government policy and terminology over the next few years. Without much doubt, however, the shift from secondary to primary care will continue, and the objectives will continue to be health focused, outcome based and consumer driven. The issues that arise from these objectives have been examined in each chapter and will remain current and relevant into the next millenium. Moreover, the major challenge for society in primary health care will remain the same, namely to provide sensitive and cost-effective care to an ageing population and to people at risk from, and with, life-style diseases. We believe that nursing in primary health care has a distinct role, not only in the delivery of care, but also in initiating, leading and evaluating changes.

References

Adcock, W. (1991) Developments in Nottingham, *Carelink* 5, London: King's Fund Centre.

Anderson, E. (1993) *Motor Neurone Disease Support Group*, London: Queens Nursing Institute Newsletter 3, 4: 7.

Anderson, J.A.D. (1969) The health team in the community, *The Lancet* 20, 7: 679–681.

Arber, S. and Gilbert, N. (1993) Men: the forgotten carers, in Bornat, J., Pereira, C., Pilgrim, D. and Williams, F. (eds) *Community Care: A Reader*, Basingstoke: Macmillan.

Arikian, V.L. (1991) Total quality management: applications to nursing service, *Journal of Nursing Administration* 21, 6: 46–50.

Armitage, S.E. (ed.) (1991) *Continuity of Nursing Care*, London: Scutari Press.

Association of Metropolitan Authorities (1994) *Local Authorities and Health Services. The Future Role of Local Authorities in the Provision of Health Services*, a discussion document, AMA.

Atkin, K. and Lunt, N. (1993) A census of direction, *Nursing Times* 89, 42: 38–41.

Atkin, K., Hirst, M., Lunt, N. and Parker, G. (1994) The role and self perceived training needs of nurses employed in general practice: observations from a national census of practice nurses in England and Wales, *Journal of Advanced Nursing* 20: 46–52.

Atkinson, F.I. (1992) Experiences of informal carers providing nursing support for disabled dependants, *Journal of Advanced Nursing* 17: 835–840.

Atkinson, J. (1987) 'I just exist'. Glasgow's single homeless men, *Community Outlook* Nov.: 12–15.

Atmarow, A., Blomfield, J. and Brady, S. (1993) The clean gang, *Nursing Times* 89(45): 30–32.

Au, W. and Au, K. (1992) *Working with Chinese Carers. A Handbook for Professionals*, London: Health Education Authority and King's Fund Centre.

Audit Commission (1985) *Managing Social Services for the Elderly More Effectively*, London: HMSO.

—— (1986) *Making a Reality of Community Care*, London: HMSO.

—— (1992) *Homeward Bound: A New Course for Community Health*, London: HMSO.

Badger, F., Cameron, E. and Evers, H. (1988) Care at the crossroads, *Health Service Journal* 98, 5,1: 1454–1455.

—— (1989) District nurses' patients – issues of caseload management, *Journal of Advanced Nursing* 14: 518–527.

Baker, V. (1994) Supporting patients with HIV, *Community Outlook* 4, 7: 19–20.

Barriball, L. and Mackenzie, A.E. (1993) Measuring the impact of nursing interventions in the community, a selective review of the literature, *Journal of Advanced Nursing* 18, 3: 401–407.

Bartlett, W. and Le Grand, J. (1994) The performance of Trusts 1994, in Robinson, R. and Le Grand, J. (eds) *Evaluating the NHS Reforms*, London: King's Fund Institute.

Batchelor, I. (1984) *Policies for a Crisis – Some Aspects of DHSS Policies for the Care of the Elderly*, London: Nuffield Provincial Hospitals Trust.

Baxter, C. (1988) Black carers in focus, *CareLink* 4: 4, London: King's Fund Centre.

Beardow, R., Oerton, J. and Victor, C. R. (1989) Evaluation of the cervical cytology screening programme in an inner city area, *British Medical Journal* 299: 98–100.

Beattie, A. (1991) Knowledge and control in health promotion: a test case for social policy and social theory, in Gabe, J, Calnan, M. and Bury, M. (eds) *The Sociology of the Health Service*, London: Routledge.

—— (1994) Healthy alliance or dangerous liaisons? The challenge of working together in health promotion, in Leathard, A. (ed.) *Going Inter-professional*, London: Routledge.

Bergen, A. (1992) Case management in community care: concepts, practices and implications for nursing, *Journal of Advanced Nursing* 17, 1106–1113.

—— (1994) Case management in the community: identifying a role for nursing, *Journal of Clinical Nursing Care* 3, 4: 251–257.

Best, G. (1989) The White Paper: challenge to local strategists, *Health Service Journal*, 8 June: 686–687.

Biggs, S. (1993) User participation and interprofessional collaboration in community care, *Journal of Interprofessional Care* 7, 2: 151–159.

Blanchard, M., Waterreus, A. and Mann, A. (1994) The nature of depression among older people in inner London and the contact with primary care, *British Journal of Psychiatry* 164: 396–402.

Bloch, D. (1975) Evaluation of nursing care in terms of process and outcome, *Nursing Research* 24,4: 256–263.

Bond, S. and Thomas, L.H. (1991) Issues in measuring outcomes of nursing, *Journal of Advanced Nursing* 16: 1492–1502.

—— (1992) Measuring patients' satisfaction with nursing care, *Journal of Advanced Nursing* 17: 52–63.

Bornat, J., Pereira, C., Pilgrim, D. and Williams, F. (eds) (1993) *Community Care: A Reader*, Basingstoke: MacMillan Press.

Bosanquet, N. (1993) Two cheers for the internal market, *Journal of Interprofessional Care* 7,2: 125–129.

Bourke-Dowling, S. (1994) Collaborative working, *Primary Health Care* 4,6: 6–8.

Bowling, A. (1981) *Delegation in General Practice. A Study of Doctors and Nurses*, London: Tavistock.

—— (1985) District Health Authority policy and the 'extended clinical role of the nurse' in primary health care, *Journal of Advanced Nursing* 10: 443–454.

Boyd, M., Brummell, K., Billingham, K. and Perkins, E.R. (1993) *The Public Health Post At Strelley: An Interim Report*, Nottingham: Nottingham Community Health NHS Trust.

Boyle, C. and Smaje, C. (1993) *Primary Health Care in London: Quantifying the Challenge*, London: King's Fund Institute.

Bradford, M. and Winn, S. (1993) A survey of practice nurses' views of health promotion, *Health Authority Journal* 52: 2.

Bradshaw, J. S. (1972) A taxonomy of social need, in McLachlan G. (ed) *Problems and Progress in Medical Care* 7th series, Oxford: Oxford University Press.

Braithwaite, V. (1992) Caregiving burden, *Research on Ageing* 14, 1: 3–27.

Brearley, S. (1990) *Patient Participation: The Literature*, Royal College of Nursing Research Series, Middlesex: Scutari Press.

British Diabetic Association (1993) *Recommendations for the Management of Diabetes in Primary Care*, London: British Diabetic Association.

British Family Heart Study (1994) Randomised controlled trial evaluating cardiovascular screening and intervention in general practice, *British Medical Journal* 308: 313–320.

Brown, K., Williams, E. and Groom, L. (1992) Health checks on patients 75 years and over in Nottinghamshire after the new contract, *British Medical Journal* 305: 619–621.

Bryar, R. (1994) An examination of the need for new nursing roles in primary health care, *Journal of Interprofessional Care* 8,1: 73–84.

Bunton, R. and Macdonald, G. (1992) *Health Promotion: Disciplines and Diversity*, London: Routledge.

Burke Masters, B. (1987) The autonomous nurse practitioner, *The Lancet* 1: 1266.

Butler, J. (1994) Origins and early development, in Robinson, R. and Le Grand, J. (eds) Evaluating the NHS Reforms, London: King's Fund Institute.

Butterworth, T. (1994) *A Delphi Survey of Optimum Practice in Nursing, Midwifery and Health Visiting*, Manchester: School of Nursing Studies, University of Manchester.

CAIPE (Centre for the Advancement of Interprofessional Education) (1992) A national survey that needs to be repeated, *Journal of Interprofessional Care* 6, 1: 65–71.

Carers' National Association (1992) *Speak up, Speak Out*, London: Carers' National Association.

—— (undated a) *Carers Code, Eight Key Principles for Health and Social Care Providers*, London: Carers' National Association.

—— (undated b) *A Fair Deal for Carers*, London: Carers' National Association.

Carpenter, G. and Demopoulos, G. (1990) Screening elderly people in the community: controlled trial of dependency surveillance using a questionnaire administered by volunteers, *British Medical Journal* 300: 1253–1256.

Carrier, J. and Kendall, I. (1995) Professionalism and interprofessionalism in health and community care: some theoretical issues, in Owens, P. and Carrier, J. *Interprofessional Issues in Community and Primary Health Care*, London: Macmillan.

Carruthers, I. (1994) Primary care-led purchasing, *King's Fund News* 17, 4: 2.

Carstairs, V. and Morris, R. (1989) Deprivation, mortality and resource allocation, *Community Medicine* 11: 364–372.

Challis, D. and Davies, B. (1986) *Case Management in Community Care: Implications for the Implementation of Caring for People*, London: King's Fund Centre.

Challis, D., Darton, R., Johnson, L., Stone, M., Traske, K. and Wall, B. (1989) *Supporting Frail Elderly People at Home: The Darlington Community Care Project*, Canterbury: Personal Social Services Research Unit: Kent University.

Challis, D., Chessum, R., Chesterman, J., Luckett, R. and Traske, K. (1990) *Case Management in Social and Health Care: The Gateshead Community Care Scheme*, Canterbury: Personal Social Services Research Unit, Kent University.

Chapman, H. (1994) Carers group, *District Nursing Association UK Newsletter* XL: 11–12.

Chew, C., Wilkin, D. and Glendinning, C. (1994) Annual assessment of patients aged 75 years and over: general practitioners' and practice nurses' views and experiences, *British Journal of General Practice* 44: 263–267.

Chisholm, J. (1990) The 1990 Contract: its history and content, *British Medical Journal* 300: 853–856.

Congress of the United States (1986) *Health Technology Case Study 37. Nurse Practitioners, Physician Assistants, and Certified Nurse-Midwives: A Policy Analysis*, Washington: Office of

Technology Assessment.

Cox, C. and Mead, A. (eds) (1975) *Sociology of Medical Practice*, London: Collier Macmillan.

Dalley, G. and Carr-Hill, R. (1991) *Pathways to Quality. A Study of Quality Management Initiatives in the NHS. A Guide for Managers*, QMI Series No 2, York: Centre for Health Economics, University of York.

Dalley, G., Baldwin, S., Carr-Hill, R., Hennessey, S. and Smedley, E. (1991) *Quality Management Initiatives in the NHS: Strategic Approaches to Improving Quality*, York: Centre for Health Economics, University of York.

Dargie, L. and Proctor, J. (1994) Setting up an arthritis clinic, *Community Outlook* 4,7: 14–17.

Davies, H. (1992) Role of the Audit Commission, *Quality in Health Care* 1 (Supplement): 528–533.

Davies, S. (1990) An approach to case finding the elderly, *Nursing Times* 86, 51: 48–51.

Day, M. (1994) Forward role?, *Nursing Times* 90, 6: 22–23.

Deming, W. (1986) *Out of Crisis*, Cambridge, MA: MIT Press.

DHSS (1976) *Priorities for Health and Social Services*, London: HMSO.

—— (1977) *Prevention and Health*, London: HMSO.

—— (1981a) *Growing Older*, Cmd. 849, London: HMSO.

—— (1981b) *The Primary Health Care Team* (Harding Report), London: HMSO.

—— (1983) *NHS Management Inquiry* (Griffiths Report), London: HMSO.

—— (1986) *Neighbourhood Nursing – A Focus for Care*, report of the community nursing review (Chairman Julia Cumberlege), London: HMSO.

—— (1987) *Promoting Better Health*, London: HMSO.

Dickinson, E. and Young, A. (1990) A framework for medical assessment of functional performance, *The Lancet* 335: 778–779.

Dickinson, E. and Mayer, P. (1995) The development and use of standardised assessment scales for elderly people. Paper given at SYSTED '94 international conference in Geneva.

Dingwall, R. (1980) Problems of teamwork in primary care, in Lonsdale, S., Webb, A. and Briggs, T. (eds) *Teamwork in the Personal Social Services and Health Care*, London: Croom Helm.

District Nursing Association (1993) *Skill Mix and GP Fundholding – Contracting Issues*, Edinburgh: DNA.

DoH (1989a) *A Strategy for Nursing: Report of the Steering Committee*, London: HMSO.

—— (1989b) *Working for Patients* Cmd.555, London: HMSO.

—— (1989c) *Caring for People: Community Care in the Next Decade and Beyond* Cmd.849, London: HMSO.

—— (1989d) *The 1990 GP Contract*, London: HMSO.

—— (1990a) *Nursing in the Community*, Report of working group (Chairman Sheila Roy), London: HMSO.

—— (1990b) *The NHS and Community Care Act*, London: HMSO.

DoH: Social Services Inspectorate (1991a) *Care Management and Assessment – A Practitioners' and Managers' Guide*, London: HMSO.

DoH (1991b) *National Health Service Management Executive Assessing Health Care Need*, London: HMSO.

—— (1992) *Health of the Nation: A Strategy for Health in England*, London: HMSO.

—— (1994a) *Developing NHS Purchasing and GP Fundholding: Towards a Primary Care Led NHS*, EL 94/79, London: DoH.

—— (1994b) *Working in Partnership: A Review of Mental Health Nursing*, London: HMSO.

Donabedian, A. (1966) Evaluating the quality of medical care, *Milbank Memorial Fund Quarterly* XLIV, 3, 2: 166–203.

Drennan, V. (1990a) Gathering information from the field, *Nursing Times* 86, 39: 46–48.

—— (1990b) Striving for fairer workloads, *Nursing Times* 86, 40: 48–49.

Ebrahim, S., Hedley, R. and Sheldon, M. (1984) Low levels of ill health among elderly nonconsulters in general practice, *British Medical Journal* 289: 1273–1275.

Edmond, E. (1993) Provision of local health education to the Asian community, *Community Outlook* 3, 7: 13–16.

Emmerson, P. (1994) Get in on the Act, *Community Outlook,* October: 15–18.

Etzioni, A. (1969) *The Semi-professions and their Organisations: Teachers, Nurses and Social Workers,* New York: The Free Press.

Evans, P. (1994) In good heart, *Community Outlook* 4,1: 31–32.

Fares, S. (1993) A smooth path home, *Nursing Times* 89, 21: 48–50.

Faugier, J. (1994) Thin on the ground, *Nursing Times* 90, 20: 64.

Ferns, T. (1994) Home mechanical ventilation in a changing health service, *Nursing Times* 90, 40: 43–45.

Freer, C. B. (1985) Geriatric screening: a reappraisal of preventive strategies in the care of the elderly, *JRCGP* 35: 288–290.

—— (1987) Detecting hidden needs in the elderly: screening or casefinding, in Taylor, R. and Buckley, E. (eds) *Preventive Care of the Elderly: A Review of Current Developments,* Royal College of General Practitioners Occasional Paper 35.

Friedson, E. (1970) *Professional Dominance,* New York: Atherton.

Gabe, J., Calnan, M. and Bury, M. (eds) *The Sociology of the Health Service,* London: Routledge.

Gibbs, I., McCaughan, D. and Griffiths, M. (1991) Skill mix in nursing: a selective review of the literature, *Journal of Advanced Nursing* 16: 242–249.

Gillam, S., Plamping, D., McClenahan, J. and Harries, J. (1994) *Community-Orientated Primary Care,* London: King's Fund Centre.

Gilmore, M., Bruce, N. and Hunt, M. (1974) *The Work of the Nursing Team in General Practice,* London: Council for the Education and Training of Health Visitors.

Glennerster, H., Matsaganis, M. and Owens, P. (1992) *A Foothold for Fundholding,* Research Report No. 12, London: King's Fund Institute.

Glennerster, H., Matsaganis, M., Owens, P. and Hancock, S. (1994) GP fundholding: wild card or winning hand?, in Robinson, R. and Le Grand, J. (eds) *Evaluating the NHS Reforms,* London: King's Fund Institute.

Graham, H. (1991) The informal sector on welfare: a crisis in caring?, *Social Science of Medicine* 32, 4: 507–515.

Green, H. (1988) *General Household Survey 1985: Informal Carers*, London: HMSO.

Gregson, B., Cartlidge, A. and Bond, J. (1991) *Interprofessional Collaboration in Primary Care Organisations*, The Royal College of Practitioners Occasional Paper 52.

Griffiths, R. (1988) *Community Care: Agenda for Action*, London: HMSO.

Gunaratnum, Y. (1993) Breaking the silence: Asian carers in Britain, in Bornat, J., Pereira, C., Pilgrim, D. and Williams, F. (eds) *Community Care: A Reader*, Basingstoke: Macmillan Press.

Handy, C. (1989) *The Age of Unreason*, London: Business Books Ltd.

Hardie, M. and Hockey, L. (eds) (1978) *Nursing Auxiliaries in Health Care*, London: Croom Helm.

Harrison, A. (1993) *Health Care UK 1992/93*, London: King's Fund Institute.

Hart, N. (1985) *The Sociology of Health and Medicine*, Ormskirk: Causeway Press.

Hart, T.J. (1983) A new type of general practitioner, *The Lancet* 2, 27–29.

Harvey, G. (1991) An evaluation of approaches to assessing the quality of nursing care using (predetermined) quality assurance tools, *Journal of Advanced Nursing* 16: 277–286.

Hearn, J. (1993) *An Exploration of Carers' Perceptions of Their Participation in the Care of Their Relatives in the Community and District Nurses' Role in this Participation*, unpublished dissertation, London: Nursing Department, King's College London.

Hearnshaw, H. M. (in press) Multi-disciplinary audit project, in Ross, F. and Elliott, M. *Innovations in Community Nursing*, Edinburgh: Community and District Nursing Association.

Henderson, J., Goldacre, M., Graveney, M. and Simmons, H. (1989) Use of medical record linkage to study readmission rates, *British Medical Journal* 299: 709–713.

Hoare, J. (1992) *Tidal Wave, New Technology Medicine and the NHS*, London: King's Fund Centre.

Hockey, L. (1972) *Use or Abuse. A Study of the State Enrolled Nurse in the Local Authority Nursing Services*, London: Queen's

Nursing Institute.

—— (1979) *Development and Progression of a Long-Term Research Programme*, unpublished PhD thesis, London: City University.

Holt, F. M. (1987) Developmental stages of the clinical nurse specialist role, *Clinical Nurse Specialist* 1: 116–118.

Horder, J. (1995) Interprofessional education for primary health and community care: present state and future needs, in Soothill, K., Mackay, L. and Webb, C. (eds) *Interprofessional Relations in Health Care*, London: Edward Arnold.

Hughes, J. (ed.) (1990) *Enhancing the Quality of Community Nursing*, London: King's Fund Centre.

Humphrey, C. and Hughes, J. (1992) *Audit and Development in Primary Care*, London: King's Fund Centre.

Humphris, D. (1994) Clinical guidelines: an industry for growth, *Nursing Times* 90, 40: 46–47.

Hunter, D. (1993) To market! To market! A new dawn for community care, *Health and Social Care* 1, 1: 3–10.

Hunter, D. and Judge, K. (1988) *Griffiths and Community Care: Meeting the Challenge*, Briefing paper no.5, King's Fund Institute.

Hutchinson, A. and Gordon, S. (1992) Primary care teamwork – making it a reality, *Journal of Interprofessional Care* 6, 1: 31–42.

Illife, S., Haines, A., Gallivan, S., Booroff, A., Goldenberg, E. and Morgan, P. (1991) Assessment of elderly people in general practice: social circumstances and mental status, *British Journal of General Practice* 41: 9–12.

Imperial Cancer Research Fund OXCHECK study group (1994) Effectiveness of health checks conducted by nurses in primary care: results of the OXCHECK study after one year, *British Medical Journal* 308: 308–312.

Irvine, D. and Irvine, S. (eds) (1991) *Making Sense of Audit*, Oxford: Radcliffe Medical Press.

James, J. (1994) Laser therapy on trial, *Primary Health Care* 4, 10: 15–20.

Jarman, B. (1983) Identification of underprivileged areas, *British Medical Journal* 286: 1705–1709.

JCAHO (1990) *Accreditation Manual for Hospitals*, Chicago: Joint Commission on Accreditation of Health Care Organisations.

Jefferies, S., McShane, S., Oerten, J., Victor, C. R. and Beardow, R. (1991) Low immunization rates in an inner city health district. Fact or fiction?, *Journal of Public Health Medicine* 13, 4: 312–317.

Jones, B. (1990) Working together: a description of residential multi-professional workshops, *Postgraduate Education for General Practice* 1: 154–159.

—— (1992) Teamwork in primary care: how much do we know about it?, *Journal of Interprofessional Care* 6, 1: 25–29.

Katz, J. and Green, E. (1992) *Managing Quality A Guide to Monitoring and Evaluating Nursing Services*, St Louis: Mosby: Year Book Inc.

Keady, J. and Nolan, M. (1994) The carer-led assessment process (CLASP): a framework for the assessment of need in dementia caregivers, *Journal of Clinical Nursing* 3: 103–108.

Kendall, S. (1993) Do health visitors promote client participation? An analysis of the health visitor–client interaction, *Journal of Clinical Nursing* 2: 103–109.

Killoran, A., Calnan, M., Cant, S. and Williams, S. (1993) Pacemaker, *Health Service Journal*, 18 Feb.: 26–27.

Kirk, R. (1992) The big picture total quality management and continuous quality improvement, *Journal of Nursing Administration* 22, 4: 24–31.

Kitson, A.L. (1986) Indicators of quality in nursing care – an alternative approach, *Journal of Advanced Nursing* 11: 133–144.

—— (1987) Raising standards of clinical practice – the fundamental issue of effective nursing practice, *Journal of Advanced Nursing* 12: 321–329.

Koch, M. W. and Fairly, T. M. (1993) *Integrated Quality Management, The Key to Improving Nursing Care Quality*, St Louis: Mosby.

Kohner, N. (1994) *Clinical Supervision in Practice*, London: King's Fund Centre.

Korczak, E. (1993) Joint assessment, *Primary Health Care* 3, 2: 8–10.

Kosberg, J. I. and Cairl, R. E. (1986) The cost of care index: a case management tool for screening informal care providers, *The Gerontologist* 26, 3: 273–278.

Latter, S., Macleod-Clark, J., Wilson-Barnett, J. and Maben, J. (1992) Health education in nursing: perceptions of practice in acute settings, *Journal of Advanced Nursing* 17: 164–172.

Leathard, A. (1994) *Going Inter-professional – Working Together for Health and Welfare*, London: Routledge.

Leedham, I. and Wistow, G. (1992) *Community Care and General Practitioners*, Nuffield Institute of Health Service Studies, Paper no. 6, University of Leeds.

Lewis, J. (1993) Community care: policy imperatives, joint planning and enabling authorities, *Journal of Interprofessional Care* 7, 1: 7–15.

Lewis, J. and Meredith, B. (1988) Daughters caring for mothers: the experience of caring and its implications for professional helpers, *Ageing and Society* 8: 1–21.

Lewis, J., Bernstock, P. and Bovell, V. (1995) The community care changes: unresolved tensions in policy and issues in implementation, *Journal of Social Policy* 24, 1: 73–94.

Lloyd, K. (1993) Community mothers' programme, *Nursing Times* 89, 26: 42–44.

London Health Consortium (1981) *Report of a Study Group of Primary Health Care in Inner London* (Acheson Report), London: DHSS.

Lonsdale, S., Webb, A., and Briggs, T. (eds) (1980) *Teamwork in the Personal Social Services and Health Care*, London: Croom Helm.

Luker, K. and Kenrick, M. (1992) An exploratory study of the sources of influence on the clinical decisions of community nurses, *Journal of Advanced Nursing* 17: 457–466.

Luski, M. (1958) *The Interdisciplinary Team, Research Methods and Problems*, National Training Laboratory: New York Press.

Luthert, J. R. and Robinson, L. (eds) (1993) *The Royal Marsden Hospital Manual of Standards of Care*, London: Blackwell Scientific Publications.

McCaffery, M. (1983) *Nursing Management of the Patient with Pain*, Philadelphia: J.B. Lippincott

McClure, L. (1984) Teamwork, myth or reality: community nurses' experience of general practice attachment, *Journal of Epidemiology and Community Health* 38,1: 68–74 and 3, 2: 9–10.

McCready, S. (1993) Audit of leg ulcers, *District Nursing Association Newsletter* 11: 2.

—— (1995) Care of leg ulcers in audit, in Ross, F. and Elliott, M. *Innovations in Community Nursing*, Edinburgh: Community and District Nursing Association UK.

McIntosh, J. (1985) District nursing: a case of political marginality, in White, R. (ed.) *Political Issues in Nursing*, Chichester: John Wiley.

McKee, M. (1993) Routine data a resource for clinical audit, *Quality in Health Care* 2: 104–111.

Mackenzie, A. E. (1989) *The Role of the District Nurse within the Community Context*, Issues in District Nursing, Paper One, Edinburgh: District Nursing Association UK.

—— (1991) *Hospital at Home*, Edinburgh: District Nursing Association UK.

—— (1992) Learning from experience in the community. An ethnographic study of district nurse students, *Journal of Advanced Nursing* 17: 682–691.

Mackenzie, A. and Cowley, S. (1993) Nursing skill-mix in the district nursing service, *District Nursing Association UK Newsletter* X,1: 1–4.

Mackenzie, A. E. and Holroyd, E. (in press) An exploration of caregiving and caring responsibilities in Chinese families, *Journal of Clinical Nursing*.

McKeown, T. (1968) Validation of screening procedures, in *Screening in Medical Care: Reviewing the Evidence*, Nuffield Provincial Hospitals Trust: Oxford University Press.

McLachlan, G. (ed.) (1972) *Problems and Progress in Medical Care*, 7th series, Oxford: Oxford University Press.

Macleod-Clark, J. (1983) Nurse–patient communication – an analysis of conversations from surgical wards, in Wilson Barnett, J. (ed.) *Nursing Research: Ten Studies in Patient Care*, Chichester:

John Wiley.

McMurray, A. (1993) *Community Health Nursing*, Melbourne: Churchill Livingstone.

Mc Naught, A. (1991) Satisfying the public and the consumer, or the public as consumer, in Mc Naught, A. (ed.) *Managing Community Health Services*: 134–149, London: Chapman and Hall.

Martin, J., Meltzer, H. and Elliot, D. (1988) *The Prevalence of Disability Amongst Adults*, OPCS, London: HMSO.

Mason, C. and Beattie, A. (1993) Nursing development unit, *Primary Health Care* 3, 9: 8–10.

Mason, G. and Webb, C. (1993) Nursing diagnosis: a review of the literature, *Journal of Clinical Nursing* 2: 67–74.

Masters, F. and Schmele, J.A. (1991) Total quality management: An idea whose time has come, *Journal of Nursing Quality Assurance* 5, 7: 7–16.

Mawby, D. (1993) Support for carers, *Nursing Times* 89, 23: 67–68.

Maxwell, R.J. (1984) Quality assessment in health, *British Medical Journal* 288: 1470–1472.

Meek, H. and Pietroni, M. (1993) Communication in cancer care – a reflective learning model using group relations methods, *Journal of Interprofessional Care* 7, 3: 229–238.

Mitchell, J. (1989) Local management in the limelight, *KF News, The Newsletter of the King's Fund* 12, 4: 3, London: King's Fund Centre.

Molde, S. and Diers, D. (1985) Nurse practitioner research: selected literature review and research agenda, *Nursing Research* 34, 6: 362–367.

Morrell, D. (1993) *Diagnosis in General Practice – Art or Science?*, London: Nuffield Provincial Hospitals Trust.

Morton, A. J. (1993) *An Exploratory Study of the Consumer's Views of Carer Support Groups*, unpublished dissertation, London: Department of Nursing, King's College London.

Morton, A.J. and Mackenzie, A.E. (1994) An exploratory study of the consumers' views of carer support groups, *Journal of Clinical Nursing* 1: 63–64.

NAHAT (National Association of Health Authorities and Trusts)

(1993) *Reinventing Healthcare Towards a New Model*, London: NAHAT.

Newman, C. (1991) Receiving patients from hospital, in Armitage, S. E. (ed.) *Continuity of Nursing Care*, London: Scutari Press.

NHSME (National Health Service Management Executive) (1991a) *Framework of Audit for Nursing Services*, London: HMSO.

—— (1991b) *Today's and Tomorrow's Priorities*, London: HMSO.

—— (1992) *The Nursing Skill Mix in the District Nursing Service*, London: HMSO.

—— (1993a) *New World New Opportunities: Nursing in Primary Health Care*, London: HMSO.

—— (1993b) *A Vision for the Future*, London: National Health Service Management Executive.

—— (undated a) *Quality in Action. The Directory*, London: National Health Service Management Executive.

—— (undated b) *Quality in Action, Worthing District Health Authority: A Case Study*, London: National Health Service Management Executive.

—— (undated c) *Measuring the Quality. Nursing Care Audit, Teaching Notes*, London: National Health Service Management Executive.

—— (undated d) *The Evolution of Clinical Audit*, London: National Health Service Management Executive.

NHSTD (National Health Service Training Directorate) (1993) *Care Management: Change Management*, Developing Managers for Community Care series, Publication no. 2160693, Bristol: NHSTD.

—— (1994) *Care Management: A Practical Development*, Developing Managers for Community Care series, Publication no. 2161194, Bristol: NHSTD.

Nolan, M. and Grant, G. (1992) Helping 'new carers' of the frail elderly patient: the challenge for nurses in acute care settings, *Journal of Clinical Nursing* 1: 303–307.

Norman, I. J. and Redfern, S. J. (1990) Measuring the quality of nursing care: a consideration of different approaches, *Journal of Advanced Nursing* 15: 1260–1271.

Novak, M. and Guest, C. (1989) Application of a multidimensional caregiver burden inventory, *The Gerontologist* 29, 6: 798–803.

Oakland, J.S. (1989) *Total Quality Management*, London: Butterworth-Heinemann.

Ochera, J., Hilton, S., Bland, J. M., Dowell, A. C. and Jones, D. R. (1993) A study of the provision of health checks and health-promotion clinics in 18 general practices, *Journal of Clinical Nursing* 2: 273–277.

Oliver, M. (1988) Flexible services, *Nursing Times* 84,14: 25–29.

OPCS (1988) Surveys of disability in Great Britain, Report 1, *The Prevalence of Disability Among Adults*, London: HMSO.

—— (1992) *OPCS Monitor. SS 92/2. General Household Survey: Carers in 1990*, London: HMSO.

Orem, D. (1985) *Nursing Concepts of Practice*, New York: McGraw-Hill.

—— (1991) (4th edn) *Nursing Concepts of Practice*, USA: Mosby Year Book.

Owens, P. and Carrier, J. (1995) *Interprofessional Issues in Community and Primary Health Care*, London: Macmillan.

Packham, S. (1993) Streetwise, *Nursing Standard* 8, 4: 18–19.

Parker, G. and Lawton, D. (1991) *Further Analysis of the 1985 General Household Survey Data on Informal Care*, Report 4, *Male Carers*, York: Social Policy Research Unit, York University.

—— (1994) *Different Types of Care, Different Types of Carer: Evidence from the General Household Survey*, London: HMSO.

Pearson, P. and Jones, K. (1994) The primary care non team?, *British Medical Journal* 309: 1387–1388.

Perkins, E. (1991) Screening elderly people: a review of the literature in the light of the new general practitioner contract, *British Journal of General Practice* 41: 382–385.

Petticrew, M., Mckee, M. and Jones, J. (1993) Coronary artery surgery: are women discriminated against?, *British Medical Journal* 306: 1164–1166

Philp, I. (1994) *Assessing Elderly People*, London: Farrand Press.

Pick, J. (1992) Assessment and care management in South Bedfordshire, *Primary Health Care Management* 2, 14: 8–10.

Pickin, C. and St Leger, S. (1993) *Assessing Health Needs Using the Life Cycle Framework*, Buckingham: Open University Press.

Pilling, S. (1994) Lifting/handling risk calculator, *Nursing Standard* 8, 35: 22–23.

Plamping, D. (1994) Community-orientated primary care: linking service development to strategic intent, *King's Fund News* 17, 1: 8.

Poulton, B. and West, M. (1994) Primary health care team effectiveness: developing a constituency approach, *Health and Social Care* 2: 77–84.

Queen's Nursing Institute (1993) *Newsletter* 4, 3, London: QNI.

Ramdas, A. (1991) Turning rhetoric into reality, *Carelink* 3, London: King's Fund Centre.

Rawson, D. (1992) The growth of health promotion theory and its rational reconstruction, in Bunton, R. and Macdonald, G. (eds) *Health Promotion: Disciplines and Diversity*, London: Routledge.

Redfern, S. J. (1993) In pursuit of quality of nursing care, *Journal of Clinical Nursing* 2: 141–148.

Redfern, S.J. and Norman, I.J. (1994) *The Validity of Quality Assessment Instruments for Nursing*, London: Nursing Research Unit, King's College London.

Reid, T. (1993) Joint input, *Nursing Times* 89, 47: 30–32.

Robinson, B.C. (1983) Validation of a caregiver strain index, *Journal of Gerontology* 38, 3: 344–348.

Robinson, J. and Yee, L. (1991) *Focus on Carers. A Practical Guide to Planning and Delivery of Community Care Services*, London: King's Fund Centre.

Robinson, R. and Le Grand, J. (eds) (1994) *Evaluating the NHS Reforms*, London: King's Fund Institute.

Roper, N., Logan, W. and Tierney, A. (1980) *The Elements of Nursing*, Edinburgh: Churchill Livingstone.

Ross, F. (1980) Primary health care in Thamesmead, *Nursing Times*, Occasional Paper 76: 18 and 19: 81–88.

—— (1988) Information sharing between patients, nurses and doctors: Evaluation of a drug guide for old people in primary health care, in Johnson, R. *Recent Advances in Nursing* 21:159–185, London: Longman.

—— (1989) Doctor, nurse and patient knowledge of prescribed medication in primary care, *Public Health* 103:131–137.

—— (1990) New horizons in community care: policy perspectives for district nursing, *Key Issues Paper No. 2*, Edinburgh: District Nursing Association.

Ross, F. and Bower, P. (1995) Standardised assessment for elderly people: a feasibility study in district nursing, *Journal of Clinical Nursing* 4: 303–310.

Ross, F. and Campbell, F. (1992) Interprofessional collaboration in the provision of aids for daily living and nursing equipment in the community – a district nurse and consumer perspective, *Journal of Interprofessional Care* 6, 2: 109–118.

Ross, F. and Elliott, M. (1995) *Innovations in Community Nursing*, Edinburgh: Community and District Nursing Association.

Ross, F. and Mackenzie, A.E. (1991) *Setting Standards for the Care of Elderly People at Home*, Report of three workshops at King's Fund Centre, Edinburgh: District Nursing Association UK.

Ross, F. and Tissier, J. (1994) *Monitoring and Action Research Project of Assessment and Care Management in Two North Battersea GP Practices*, unpublished research report, St George's Hospital Medical School.

—— (1995) Health promotion education for the primary health care team – is current provision adequate for future challenges?, *Journal of Interprofessional Care* 9 (2): 139–149.

Ross, F. M., Bower, P. J. and Sibbald, B. S.(1994) Practice nurses: characteristics, workload and training needs, *British Journal of General Practice* 44: 15–18.

Roy, S. (Chairman) (1990) Report of the working group, *Nursing in the Community*, London: HMSO.

RCGP (Royal College of General Practitioners) (1972) *The Future General Practitioner – Learning and Teaching*, London: British Medical Journal.

RCGP (1985) What sort of doctor?, Report from *General Practice* 23, London: RCGP.

Royal College of Nursing (1989) *A Framework for Quality. Royal College of Nursing Standards of Care Project*, London: Royal College of Nursing.

Royal College of Physicians and British Geriatrics Society (1992) *Standardised Assessment Scales for Elderly People (SAFE)*, London: Royal College of Physicians of London.

Royal Commission on the National Health Service (1979) *Merrison Report*, London: HMSO.

Rutgers, M.J. and Berkel, H. (1990) Short communication, new concepts in health care: some preliminary ideas, *International Journal of Health Planning and Management* 5: 215–220.

Salvage, J. (1990) The importance of nursing, *KF News. The Newsletter of the King's Fund* 13, 4: 1, London: King's Fund Centre.

—— (ed.) (1991) *Nurse Practitioners. Working for Change in Primary Health Care Nursing*, London: King's Fund Centre.

Saunders, D., Coulter, A. and McPherson, K. (1989) *Varieties in Hospital Admission Rates: A Review of the Literature*, London: King's Fund Centre.

Savill, R. and Bartholomew, J. (1994) Planning better discharges, *Journal of Community Nursing* 8, 3: 10–16.

Schon, D. A. (1987) *Educating the Reflective Practitioner*, San Francisco: Jossey Bass.

—— (1992) The crisis of professional knowledge and the pursuit of an epistemiology of practice, *Journal of Interprofessional Care* 6, 1: 49–63.

SETRHA (South East Thames Regional Health Authority) (1983) *Nursing in South East Thames Nurse Practitioner Projects 1992–1994*, Bexhill-on-Sea: SETRHA.

Shaw, G.B. (1911) *The Doctor's Dilemma*, Harmondsworth: Penguin.

Shaw, S. M. (1984) Measurement of health outcomes, *The New Zealand Nursing Journal* 77: 26–27.

Simoyi, P. (1993) Dialysis in the community, *Community Outlook* 3, 9: 37–38.

Skeet, M. (1978) Division of labour roles, responsibility and accountability within the team concept, in Hardie, M. and Hockey, L. (eds) *Nursing Auxiliaries in Health Care*, London: Croom Helm.

Smith, P., Mackintosh, M. and Towers, B. (1993) Implications of the new NHS contracting system for the district nursing service in one health authority: a pilot study, *Journal of Interprofessional Care* 7, 2: 115–124.

Soothill, K., MacKay, L. and Webb, C. (eds) *Interprofessional Relations in Health Care*, London: Edward Arnold.

South East London Screening study group (1977) A randomized controlled trial of multiphasic screening: results of the South-East London screening study, *International Journal of Epidemiology* 6: 357–360.

Spitzer, W. O., Sackett, D. L. and Sibley, J.C. (1974) The Burlington randomised trial of the nurse practitioner, *New England Journal of Medicine* 290, 5: 251–256.

Spratley, J. (1989) *Disease Prevention and Health Promotion in Primary Health Care*, London: Health Education Authority.

Stevens, A. and Raferty, J. (1994) Introduction in Stevens, A. and Raferty, J. *Health Care Needs Assessment,* Oxford: Radcliffe.

Stilwell, B. (1984) The nurse in practice, *Nursing Mirror*, 158, 21: 17–19.

—— (1991) The rise of the practice nurse, *Nursing Times* 87, 24: 26–28.

Stilwell, B., Greenfield, S., Drury, M. and Hull, F.M. (1987) A nurse practitioner in general practice: working style and pattern of consultations, *Journal of the Royal College of General Practitioners* 37: 154–157.

St Leger, S., Shneiden, H., and Walsworth-Bell, J. P. (1992) *Evaluating Health Services' Effectiveness,* Buckingham: Open University Press.

Stone, P. (1994) Nurse practitioners' research review: quality of care, *Nurse Practitioner*, June, 7: 21, 27.

Storrie, J. (1992) Mastering interprofessionalism – an enquiry into the development of Masters' programmes with an interprofessional focus, *Journal of Interprofessional Care* 6, 3: 253–261.

Syred, M. (1981) The abdication of the role of health education by hospital nurses, *Journal of Advanced Nursing* 6: 27–33.

Talbot, R. (1991) Underprivileged areas and health care planning: implications of use of Jarman indicators of urban deprivation, *British Medical Journal* 302: 383–386.

Tannahill, A. (1992) Epidemiology and health promotion: a common understanding, in Bunton, R. and MacDonnald, G. (eds) *Health Promotion: Disciplines and Diversity*, London: Routledge.

Taylor, R. and Buckley, E. (eds) *Preventive Care of the Elderly: A Review of Current Developments*, Royal College of General Practitioners Occasional Paper 35.

Thomas, R. and Corney, R. (1993) The role of the practice nurse in mental health, *Journal of Mental Health* 2: 65–72.

Thomas, S. (1993a) Health promotion programme, *Nursing Times* 89, 23: 63–67.

—— (1993b) *Intensive Care at Home*, Edinburgh: District Nursing Association UK.

Tierney, A., Worth, A., Closs, S., King, C. and Macmillan, M. (1994) Older patients' experiences of discharge from hospital, *Nursing Times* 90, 21: 36–39.

Tones, B.K. (1983) Education and health promotion: new directions, *Journal of the Institute for Health Education* 21, 4: 121–129.

—— (1986) Health education and the ideology of health promotion: a review of alternative approaches, *Health Education Research* 1: 3–12.

Touche Ross Management Consultants (1994) *Evaluation of Nurse Practitioner Pilot Projects. Summary Report*, Surrey: NHS Management Executive, South Thames.

Townsend, P. and Wedderburn, D. (1965) The aged in the welfare state, *Occasional Papers in Social Administration* No.14, London: Bell.

Townsend, P., Phillimore, P. and Beattie, A. (1988) *Health and Deprivation: Inequality and the North*, London: Croom Helm.

Traynor, M. (1994) The views and values of community nurses and their managers: research in progress, *Journal of Advanced Nursing* 20: 101–109.

Tremellen, J. (1992) Assessment of patients aged over 75 years in general practice, *British Medical Journal* 305: 621–624.

Tremellen, J. and Jones, D. (1989) Attitudes and practices of the primary health care team towards assessing the very elderly, *Journal of The Royal College of General Practitioners* 39: 142–144.

Trent Health (1993) *Focus on Asthma, an Aid to Contracting*, Sheffield: Trent Health Region.

Trnobranski, P.H. (1994) Nurse practitioner: redefining the role of the community nurse?, *Journal of Advanced Nursing* 19: 134–139.

Tudor Hart, J. (1983) A new type of general practitioner, *The Lancet* 2: 27–29.

Turton, P. (1983) Health education and the district nurse, *Nursing Times Community Outlook* 79, 32: 222–229.

Twigg, J. (1989) Models of carers: how do social care agencies conceptualise their relationship with informal carers?, *Journal of Social Policy* 18, 1: 53–66.

—— (ed.) (1992) *Carers Research and Practice*, London: HMSO.

—— (1993) Integrating carers into the service system: six strategic responses, *Ageing and Society* 13: 141–170.

Twigg, J. and Atkin, K. (1994) *Carers Perceived: Policy and Practices in Informal Care*, Milton Keynes: Open University Press.

Twigg, J., Atkin, K. and Perring, C. (1990) *Carers and Services: A Review of Research*, London: HMSO.

Twinn, S.F. (1989) *Change and Conflict in Health Visiting Practice: Dilemmas in Assessing the Professional Competence of Health Visitor Students*, unpublished PhD thesis, London: University of London, Institute of Education.

UK Clearing House (1993) *Outcomes Briefing*, introductory issue, Spring, Leeds: Nuffield Institute for Health.

UKCC (1991) *Report on Proposal for the Future of Community Education and Practice. Post Registration Education and Practice Project*, London: United Kingdom Central Council.

—— (1992) *The Scope of Professional Practice*, London: United Kingdom Central Council.

—— (1994) *The Future of Professional Practice – the Council's Standards for Education and Practice following Registration*, London: United Kingdom Central Council.

—— (1995) *Clinical Supervision. An Initial Position Statement*, London: United Kingdom Central Council.

Ungerson, C. (1993) Caring and citizenship: a complex relationship, in Bornat, J., Pereira, C., Pilgrim, D. and Williams, F. (eds)

Community Care, a Reader: 143–151, Basingstoke: Macmillan.

Usherwood, T. (1993) The primary care organisation: team or hologram?, *Journal of Interprofessional Care* 7, 3: 211–216.

Vaughan, B . (1994) What drives the change: A nursing perspective, *King's Fund News* 17, 1: 1–2.

Victor, C. R. (1991) *Health and Health Care in Later Life*, Milton Keynes: Open University Press.

Victor, C. R. and Lamping, D. (1994) Is mortality a good proxy measure of morbidity?, paper presented at Faculty of Public Health Medicine, Summer Conference, July 1994, London.

Victor, C. and Vetter, N. (1985) The early readmission of the elderly to hospital, *Age and Ageing* 14: 37–42.

—— (1988) Preparing the elderly for discharge from hospital: a neglected aspect of patient care?, *Age and Ageing* 17: 155–163.

Victor, C. R., Nazareth, B., Hudson, M. and Fuloph, N. (1993) The inappropriate use of hospital beds in an inner London DHA, *Health Trends* 25, 3: 94–97.

Vitaliano, P., Young, H. and Russo, J. (1991) Burden: a review of measures used among caregivers of individuals with dementia, *The Gerontologist* 31, 1: 67–75.

Wade, B. (1993) The job satisfaction of health visitors, district nurses and practice nurses working in areas served by four trusts: year 1, *Journal of Advanced Nursing* 18: 992–1004.

Walker, J. (1994) Caring for elderly people with persistent pain in the community: a qualitative perspective on attitudes of patients and nurses, *Health and Social Care* 2: 221–228.

Walker, L. (1992) *The Alloa Continence Centre*, Queen's Nursing Institute Newsletter (Scotland, December), Edinburgh: QNI.

Webb, A.L. and Hobdell, M. (1980) Co-ordination and teamwork in the health and personal social services, in Lonsdale, S. (ed.) *Teamwork in the Personal Social Services and Health Care*, London: Croom Helm.

White, R. (ed.) (1985) *Political Issues in Nursing*, Chichester: John Wiley & Sons.

WHO (World Health Organisation) (1978a) *Alma Ata Declaration*, Copenhagen: WHO Regional Office for Europe.

—— (1978b) *Primary Health Care*, Geneva: WHO and UNICEF.

—— (1986) *Ottowa Charter for Health Promotion*, Geneva: World Health Organisation.

—— (1989) Working Group, Regional Office for Europe, The Principles of Quality Assurance, *Quality Assurance in Health Care* 1, 2/3: 79–95.

Wilkin, D., Hallam, L. and Doggett, M. (1992) *Measures of Need and Outcome for Primary Health Care*, Oxford: Oxford University Press.

Williams, I. (1992) *Do Health Checks Work? Over 75 Care and Assessment and Health Promotion*, Oxford: Radcliffe Medical Press.

Williams, I. and Fitton, F. (1988) Factors affecting early unplanned readmission of elderly patients to hospital, *British Medical Journal* 297: 784–787.

—— (1991) Use of nursing and social services by elderly patients discharged from hospital, *British Journal of General Practice* 41: 72–75.

Williams, I. and Wallace, P. (1993) *Health Checks for People Aged 75 Years and Over*, Royal College of General Practitioners, Occasional paper no. 59.

Williams, S.J., Calnan, M., Cant, S.L. and Coyle, J. (1993) All change in the NHS? Implications of the NHS reforms for primary care prevention, *Sociology of Health and Illness, A Journal of Medical Sociology* 15, 1: 43–67.

Williamson, J., Stokoe, I., Grays, S. and Fisher, M. (1964) Old people at home: their unreported needs, *The Lancet* 1: 117–120.

Wilson, C. (1987) *Hospital Wide Quality Assurance: Models for Implementation and Development*, Ontario: W.B. Saunders.

Wilson, C. and Bannister, A. (1989) District nursing: the Preston way, *Carelink* No.7.

Wilson Barnett, J. (ed.) (1983) *Nursing Research: Ten Studies in Patient Care*, Chichester: John Wiley.

Woods, J., Patten, M. and Reilly, P. (1983) Primary care teams and the elderly in Northern Ireland, *Journal of the Royal College of General Practitioners* 33: 693–697.

Working Party on Clinical Guidelines in Palliative Care (1994) *Guidelines for Managing Cancer Pain in Adults*, London: National Council for Hospice and Specialist Palliative Care Services.

Young, K. and Haynes, R. (1993) Assessing population needs in primary health care: the problem of GP attachment, *Journal of Interprofessional Care* 7,1: 15–27.

Zarit, S.H. (1989) Editorial – Do we need another "stress and caregiving" study?, *The Gerontologist* 29, 2: 147–148.

Zola, I. (1975) Medicine as an institution of social control, in Cox, C. and Mead, A. (eds) *Sociology of Medical Practice*, London: Collier Macmillan.

Index

Printed in the United States
by Baker & Taylor Publisher Services